MW01250746

Personal Training Log

Book # _____

Start Date _____ Finish _____

PERSONAL INFORMATION

NAME_____

ADDRESS_____

CITY_____ POSTAL CODE _____

TEL_____

EMERGENCY INFORMATION

NAME_____

ADDRESS_____

RELATION_____ TEL _____

DOCTOR _____

DOCTOR'S PHONE _____

MEDICAL INFO(allergies etc) _____

_____

_____

K & KB ENTERPRISES

For information regarding permission, write to:

K & K.B Enterprises
829 Norwest Road, Unit 711,
Kingston, Ontario, K7P 2N3
CANADA
Tel: 613-532-9117

For more information visit us on-line at **www.ptlogit.com**

ISBN 0-9688533-1-5

Designed, printed and bound in Canada by
        Your Choice Communications
        20 Slader Heights Street ✦ Ajax, Ontario L1Z 1P8
        Phone: 416-558-1154 ✦ www.yourchoicecom.com
        Special thanks to the team of Brian & Nesrin

Cover design & page layout by Nesrin Genc
(Your Choice Communications)

Web design for PTL by: Jared Cole
jaredcole23@hotmail.com

Forward

Having known Lou Bilkovski as a personal friend for over 25 years, I can say he is a man of passion. Passion for achieving his dreams and in the process aiding others in achieving theirs.

As a police officer, Lou has always striven to maintain a level of physical excellence and performed his duty of serving and protecting the public with pride - a pride he continues to exuberate in everything he takes on.

It was this knowledge of Lou's loyalty to people, pride in performance, work ethics and personal passion that made me select him to lead the Anti-Doping Unit (the first in Canada) for Neutron Fitness & Sports Organization. As president of Neutron, an Organization that promotes drug-free bodybuilding, fitness, figure and sports athletic competitions, I required the professionalism and integrity of someone that believed as strongly as I did in the value of positive role models and leading a healthy, drug-free lifestyle. Lou is that man. Lou has been conducting drug testing for the CCES (Canadian Centre of Ethics in Sports) and at all Neutron events since 1999 and is one of only 80 certified Doping Control Officers in Canada.

I also know of Lou's love and passion for Football. He has been actively coaching High school Football for over 16 years with a focus on strength and conditioning techniques. His love for working with kids is evident in the founding of the Ontario Provincial Police Minor Football League for youth ages 11-13 years.

Lou continues to train and motivate others. As a personal trainer he focuses on each client bringing out their strengths and improving on their weaknesses. He is inspired each time he helps bring a dream to reality through proper goal setting and guidance.

Lou created the P.T.L. (Personal Training Log) to help give the edge to those who are seeking improved levels of health and fitness. The P.T.L. was designed to assist you in setting, tracking and maintaining your goals regardless of what sport you enjoy or what level of fitness you are presently at.

Lou understands the vital importance goal setting and tracking plays in achieving success and he wants to share this knowledge with you. Experience the satisfaction of reaching your goals and dreams and feel the passion that Lou has experienced from utilizing the tools provided in the P.T.L.

I wholeheartedly endorse Lou's book and wish you the very best on your journey to improved longevity.

Stay Strong!

Stephen C. Mackey H.G.F.N.
President
Neutron Fitness & Sports Organization
International Fitness Sanctioning Body for Canada
Ms. Fitness Canada & Ms. International Fitness Canada
www.neutronsports.com

Acknowledgment

Congratulations! You are well on your way to developing the best from within and The Personal Training Log is key for you to reach your goals. The PTL will assist you to:

o   Stay physically active.

o   Maintain excellent overall health both physically and mentally.

o   Believe in yourself and desire to make the personal changes that will lead to a healthier lifestyle.

o   Challenge yourself and understand the importance of tracking your progress.

o   Compete for the first time in any sports area be it natural bodybuilding, fitness, fitness model, figure or other sports athletics competitions.

My name is Sandra Mackey; I am the Executive Vice President for Neutron Fitness & Sports Organization, the International Fitness Sanctioning Body for Canada and a contributing Writer for Ms. Fitness Magazine.

Neutron Fitness & Sports Organization was developed in 1998 as a counter-response to increasing steroid and drug use among competitive athletes in Canada and around the world. Neutron was the first organization to introduce an anti-doping unit to the Natural Sports Movement.

The focus of Neutron Sports is to educate and support the promotion of drug-free sporting events by providing a drug-free platform in which natural athletes can compete. Education on the benefits of competing drug-free is the key to our success and our athletes are the positive role models that we promote to our communities. The essence of fair play, integrity, honesty and respect all point to the importance of being clean and being your best, naturally. Neutron plays a vital role in the establishment of ethics and sportsmanship that is sadly lacking in today's competitive sports.

Drug usage associated with strength training and bodybuilding is incongruous to good health and negates the essence of sportsmanship and the true spirit of athletics.

In order for an athlete to get the "competitive edge" naturally, requires a complete and detailed guide so that you can track every step of your journey to the very smallest detail. The PTL gives you the tools you need to be able to focus on those areas in which you are excelling and those you need to adjust or improve on.

Neutron is very serious about its Drug-Free Policy and calls upon CCES (Canadian Centre for Ethics in Sport) to ensure the athletes that compete in a Neutron Event are drug-free. With the support of CCES, Neutron promotes ethical bodybuilding, fitness and natural sporting competitions in Canada. All drug testing is done to I.O.C. (International Olympic Committee) standards. Random testing is done throughout the year to any members of Neutron as well as at all Neutron events.

Neutron promotes ethical conduct in all aspects of sport and is committed to promoting a fair and drug-free environment for all athletes. Here, athletes can share in a sport system in which hard earned efforts of training, determination and discipline on a fair and even playing field can be displayed.

Respect is paramount with Neutron. All athletes are treated like family where they can compete with pride as friendships are made in their pursuit of athletic excellence.

The Personal Training Log is an exceptional tool that can and will assist you in achieving your goals; be it to compete in an event or to achieve the ultimate physical state of exceptional health and fitness.

Today I challenge you to challenge yourself. Make the most out of life and treat your health and your body with the respect it deserves. Be a role model for the future generation of athletes and train naturally, becoming the very best you can, through proper training and hard work.

One day you may take the stage and inspire others to follow in your foot steps to exceptional health and fitness. You're well on your way…with the Personal Training Log as your guide!

For more information on Neutron Fitness and Sports Organization, visit our website at www.neutronsports.com or call (905) 723-1551 or email drugfree@neutronsports.com

Stay Strong!

Sincerely,

Sandra M. Mackey RNCP H.G.F.N.
Executive Vice President
Neutron Fitness & Sports Organization
International Fitness Sanctioning Body for Canada
Contributing Writer for Ms. Fitness Magazine
www.neutronsports.com
drugfree@neutronsports.com
(905) 723-1551
"Serving you with Integrity & Honour"

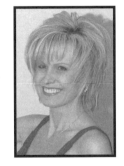

Contents

Enter Cycle 1
    The Personal Trainers Corner
    Photograph – Start
    Photograph – End of Cycle 1
    Workout & Nutrition Log Sheets

Enter Cycle 2
    The Personal Trainers Corner
    Photograph – End of Cycle 1
    Photograph – End of Cycle 2
    Workout & Nutrition Log Sheets

Enter Cycle 3
    The Personal Trainers Corner
    Photograph – End of Cycle 2
    Photograph – End of Cycle 3
    Workout & Nutritional Log Sheets

Introduction

Welcome to PTL – The Personal Training Log – Third Edition. You may not realize this, but you really have taken one of the most important steps to getting yourself in great shape.

By maintaining a training log, you will undoubtedly reach your fitness goals far quicker than without one and at the same time, you will substantially reduce the chance of quitting your fitness routine due to motivation.

I've listened to many people, young and old tell me how they just want to go to the gym and not worry about logging information. I will never understand this mentality. How do they remember what weight they used the day before or the week before? Do they just go to the gym and repeat the exact same weight for the exact same repetitions? How do they learn what is working for them and what isn't? This is not progress, this is just going through the motions and that's it. I've never lived my life this way and I don't exercise this way either.

Regardless of your age or level of fitness, the same factors affect your progress. These factors include your daily nutritional intake, your sleep, frequency between workouts, frequency between aerobic workouts, the time you workout each day and the intensity of your workouts. Each of these factors are tracked daily in PTL – The Personal Training Log – Second Edition. But there's more, the PTL also allows you to track before and after photo's of yourself, up to two cardio sessions per day plus a fitness class of your choice such as Yoga, Pilates, Spin or what ever you choose, there is also a place for you to tally all the calories you have burned and compare it to what you took in that day. There is also a spot for you to track changes in your body measurements and strength increases.

The PTL is designed to keep you organized and motivated to challenge yourself each and every time you go into the gym.

Enjoy!

Using The Personal Training Log (P.T.L.)

The PTL is a twelve (12) week daily personal training log that is broken up into three cycles made up of four weeks in each. It is designed to not only track your weight training sessions but up to two aerobic sessions per day, any fitness class you may take, your daily sleep, abdominal training, your tempo on each set you complete, your total calories burned in a day and your daily nutritional intake. All this information is provided to you at a glance, which will help you to assess where you may need to improve and make changes.

The PTL is simple to use and much of the information you enter is self-explanatory. However, the proceeding pages will explain how to use the PTL so you can get the most out of it.

Phase

When you turn to the weight lifting recording pages you will notice at the top that there is a space for the date. After the date you will see the word "Phase". This area allows persons that utilize a Periodized training method to record what Phase they are training in.

Periodization training is just as it suggests, during each period of your training you are focusing on a certain aspect. For instance, during one Phase of your training you may be focusing on Toning, on your next Phase you may be focusing on Strength. This area allows you to record and see the Phase you are in at a glance.

As an assistant Strength and Conditioning Coach for the Queen's University Golden Gaels Football Team, this method of training is imperative. The only difference is we utilize different phases that are specific to improving sports performance.

Day

You will also notice at the top of the workout pages that the word "Day" appears. On this line you simply write down which body part you intend to train that session, an example of this would be for you to write "Chest/Back. This means you will be training your Chest and your Back this session. This will allow you to see at a glance what you were training on that particular day.

Set

The word "Set" represents the amount of times you will be performing a prescribed number of repetitions. For example, if you plan to do 10 repetitions of a prescribed weight on the Leg Press, once you complete all 10 consecutive repetitions, this would represent 1 set.

Reps

The word "Reps" is the short form for repetitions. This is the amount of times you will be lifting a prescribed weight consecutively. Therefore, when you see 3 x 10. This represents 3 sets of 10 repetitions, with a certain amount of weight for each set.

"Tempo"

"Tempo" is a key word in weight lifting today and one that you will not hear from most people working out in a gym. However, ask a personal trainer and he or she will tell you it is another key element to consider when you are weight training.

Depending on what your goals are for training, you must manipulate different elements in your training to stimulate progress. Elements such as the number of sets you do, the amount of repetitions, the amount of time you rest between each of your sets and "Tempo" all play key roles in your progress.

"Tempo" simply refers to the time it takes to do one complete repetition in a particular exercise. "Tempo" is made up of a three-digit number that tells you how long to take to bring a weight down, pause at the bottom and then raise the weight up. For example, if you are bench pressing, you may see a "Tempo" rate of 3-1-2. This means you will bring the weight down (eccentric movement) for a count of three seconds, hold it at the bottom for a count of one second and then raise it (concentric movement) for a count of two seconds. Following this approach, it would mean that each repetition would take you 6 seconds to complete.

By simply manipulating your "Tempo" you can give yourself a completely different workout and force your body to respond to a different stimulus and therefore make gains in your strength, stamina or power.

As a general rule of thumb, a faster "Tempo" is used to develop power and explosive strength. A slower "Tempo" is usually used to build size.

Cardio Session #1 and #2:

The PTL provides for the recording of two aerobic sessions per day. These two sections will be of interest to anyone wishing to accelerate the fat burning process by completing two aerobic sessions in the same day.

Research has shown that it is far more beneficial to complete two shorter but separate cardio sessions than one longer session.

New to this section is **Activity Pulse Rate, Recovery Pulse Rate** and **Difference**. This area now lets you record your Activity Pulse Rate, which is taken immediately after you complete your cardio training. The Recovery Pulse Rate is taken two (2) minutes after you complete your cardio training and the Difference is Activity Pulse Rate subtracted by Recovery Pulse Rate. As you get in better cardiovascular shape the Difference will become a higher number.

So what are normal pulse rates? Well for an adult it is anywhere between 60 and 100 beats, while well conditioned athletes can have a resting heart rate between 40 and 60 beats per minute.

The first thing you are going to need to know is your Resting Heart Rate. Make sure you are relaxed and have been sitting for five minutes, take your left middle finger and index finger and place it on your carotid artery, which is found on the side of your neck. Make sure you have found your pulse and then start counting for 10 seconds, take this number and multiply it by six. This will give you your Resting Heart Rate.

The formula for determining your maximum heart rate is 220 minus your age. Your target heart rate during or just after exercise should be 60 to 80 percent of this. Therefore, if you are 50 years old, take 220 minus 50 = 170, now take 60 to 80 percent of this number which is 102 – 136 beats per minute is the zone you want to be in.

You should start to see a positive change in recovery in approximately 4 weeks! This section is located on the weight lifting recording pages under the two cardio sessions provided per day.

Fitness Class:

This is another new feature to the PTL. It is located on each of the weight lifting pages and allows you to record and keep track of any fitness class you take, whether it's a Spin Class, Pilates, Yoga or what ever, you can now keep track of this class.

Daily Sleep Tracker:

Sleep plays a very significant role in performance and growth. This is when your body has the greatest chance to repair itself from the workout which tears down your muscle. It is through proper nutrition and sleep that the body can repair it self and grow bigger and stronger. Do not neglect getting enough sleep.

This section lets you record the time you go to bed and the time you get up. It also provides an area for "comments" which is very important. This is such a simple section but provides a great deal of information as to why one is not performing up to a certain level. Let's say you enter 10 p.m. as the time you go to bed and wake up at 7:00 a.m. This represents 9 hours of sleep, which means you should be ready to go come morning. But your kids are sick with a cold and you had to get up three times during the night. This explanation should be entered into the "comments" area and can explain why your performance in the gym was not up to par.

Daily Ab Tracker:

If any of you are like myself and neglected to do your abs because you left them at the end of your workout and you now have no time to do them. You will understand why this section was made to stand- alone. I found by making it a separate section I no longer neglected to do my "abs". I just didn't want to see this area left blank every workout. I now always perform at least two abdominal exercises per session. It worked for me. I hope it will work for you.

The Daily Nutrition Tracker:

As you have probably already flipped through the pages, you will have noticed that the PTL provides you with a daily nutritional tracking system. It provides space for you to record up to six meals a day. I suggest you obtain a good calorie counter book that will display the nutritional content of all types of foods including fast food restaurants. To obtain the most benefit of this feature, simply enter everything you consume in a day and enter the time you consumed it.

You are provided three (3) options in the manner in which you may track your meals. The first is by writing down your meals and entering the total calories for each. At the end of the day just add up your calories.

The second option is for those of you that are counting points for everything you consume. If any of you are utilizing a program that assigns points to your food you can now write down your meals and the corresponding points for each in the space provided. There is also a space for you to enter your "Target Number of Points" for the day. At the end of the day you can then subtract your target points from your actual points and write down the difference in a plus or minus number in the space provided so that you can see in a glance how you did that day.

The third and final option is to track your meals by grams. This method allows you to see exactly the type of calories you are consuming at each meal.

At the end of your day, simply tally your total grams for each category protein, fat and carbohydrates. To obtain your total calories for each, use the following formula:

Multiply total grams of Protein X 4 = Protein Calories
Multiply total grams of Carbs   X 4 = Carbohydrate Calories
Multiply total grams of Fat   X 9 = Fat Calories

Add all three of these totals and enter the grand total in the "Total Calories" box. To obtain your daily percentage of each nutrient, simply divide the total calories of each nutrient by the "Total Calories" and enter the percentages under each area.

At the bottom of this page you will find a line for you to enter your Total Calories Consumed and another line for Total Calories Burned. The Total Calories Burned can be carried over from the weight lifting page that tally's all your Cardio workouts for the day.

Take this total and subtract it from you total calories consumed. This will give you an idea of how many calories you are consuming versus how many calories you are expending.

Keep in mind that the Total Calories Burned for the day does not take into account any other activities you do. That means, every thing from watching T.V., driving a car to just breathing, you are burning calories. There are various websites that will give you this information, just search "estimate calories burned for various activities". This system is not totally accurate, but you will be able to get a reasonable picture of how you are doing.

There is also an area for you to track your "Water." Many people today lack enough water in their diet. It truly is a key element to good health and weight loss! Try to take in water with all your meals. I have moved this section to each of the six Meal Headings so as to encourage you to drink water with all your meals. You will notice the heading "Meal 1" then you will see "Time" enter the time you eat in the space provided. Just after that you will see H2O and a space for you to track how many cups or litres of water you consumed with your meal!

Progress Report

The Progress Report is a single page that is broken up into two areas, "Measurements" and "Strength." In the "measurements" area, simply take your measurements for each of the specified body parts and enter the values under "Start." Once you have done this, think about what you would like to achieve. For example, your "Start" measurement for your waist may be 46". You could set a realistic goal of 43" to be attained by the end of the third cycle. To help motivate you along the way, enter your measurements after completing each four- week cycle. At the end of 12 weeks subtract your "goal" measurement from your "start measure-ment to see the difference.

In the Progress Report there is a measurement for Hip-to-Waist ratio. This measurement is new to the PTL. According to current medical research this is a better predictor of the risk of heart attack rather than body-mass index (BMI), which is the current standard.

BMI is based on height and weight, it does not take into account how muscular a person is.

Research has shown that having a potbelly is a better predictor of heart trouble rather than weight alone.

Waist-to-Hip Ratio is calculated by dividing your waist measurement by your hip measurement. Your hips are the widest part of your buttocks. Your goal if you are a man should be to have a Waist-to-Hip Ratio of 0.95 or less. For a woman your Waist-to-Hip Ratio should be 0.8 or less.

In the "Strength Report" you have the opportunity to set strength increases for yourself in 10 different exercises. For example, the most common assessment of strength is in the bench press. Simply take the maximum weight you can lift for one repetition and enter this amount under "Start" then set your "goal".

Track your progress to your goal by doing an assessment after each "Cycle". You will find that there is a direct correlation between strength and size. As your muscles get bigger your strength goes up.

Photographs

You will find pages marked "Photograph – Start", "Photograph End of Cycle 1" "Photograph End of Cycle 2", "Photograph End of Cycle 3". These pages have been provided for you so that you may take full body pictures of yourself and evaluate your progress. Enter a photo of yourself on the pages provided after each cycle. Do not neglect this feature, it will be of great value to you motivationally and eventually you will become inspirational to others. Once you have made the changes to your body, believe me, you will want to show your before and after photographs, that represents your hard work and perseverance.

Personal Fitness Evaluation

This section is made up of two pages and can be found at the beginning of each cycle. It is imperative that you take the time to fill out this area. Here is where you will have the opportunity to write down your goals and set up your fitness plan for the cycle. Remember, when you write out your goals and fitness plan, it reaffirms your commitment to them and paints a clear picture of where you are heading and how you are going to get there.

This section also provides a battery of tests so that you will be able to see your current fitness level. The tests can be done on your own or through a personal trainer. If you are new to fitness, it would be wise to utilize a personal trainer who would be able to assess your results and make worthwhile lifestyle changes with you.

Once you finish each of the cycles you will find a single page called the Progress Evaluation page. This page compliments the Personal Fitness Evaluation pages by asking you a few simple questions such as "did you meet your goals for this cycle?" If you did, great, but if you ran into a few bumps it asks you to write down what they were and what you can do to improve during the next cycle.

This single page just ties everything together and lets you write down what you already know. If for some reason you did not meet all your goals during the cycle, don't view that as a negative. Just the simple fact that you are taking the time to think about your current fitness level and some of the lifestyle changes you want to make is positive in itself. Reassess your goals and make smaller ones next time. Don't try to change your lifestyle to drastically, you took years to develop your current lifestyle, trying to change it overnight is a recipe for disaster. Take your time and make small changes you can live with, make it fun for yourself. Don't treat fitness as a chore, rather see it for what it is, time for yourself.

Remember; the Personal Fitness Evaluation page is at the beginning of each cycle and the Progress Evaluation page is at the end of each cycle.

Supplement and Medication Tracker

This chart can be found on page 11. It is a single page that lets you track any type of medication you have been prescribed or supplements you are taking. It simply lets you know at a glance when you started a particular medication or supplement and when you stopped using it.

To use this section simply put down the supplement or medication on the left hand side, the months are provided with 3 boxes allotted for each month. Each box represents approximately 10 days. In the boxes enter the day you started taking your supplement/medication, for example if you start taking a Whey Protein on the 12th of June, just place the number 12 in the second box for the month of June. Now, lets say you stop taking this protein on the 04th of September. All you would do is enter 04 in the first box under September; you could then highlight the area from the 12th of June to the 04th of September.

If you stop using Whey Protein for a while and then start up again on the 26th of November again just place the number 26 under the 3rd box of November. This section is very simple to use and extremely informative.

You can track up to 28 different supplements/medications!

Supplements or Medications	JAN	FEB	MAR	APR	MAY	JUN	JUL	AUG	SEPT	OCT	NOV	DEC
Ex. Protein - Ultra Whey	2				1				5			
Ex. Creatine - ABC Brand				7		4	9				2	8
1.												
2.												
3.												
4.												
5.												
6.												
7.												
8.												
9.												
10.												
11.												
12.												
13.												
14.												
15.												
16.												
17.												
18.												
19.												
20.												
21.												
22.												
23.												
24.												
25.												
26.												
27.												
28.												

Example of Workout Log Sheet

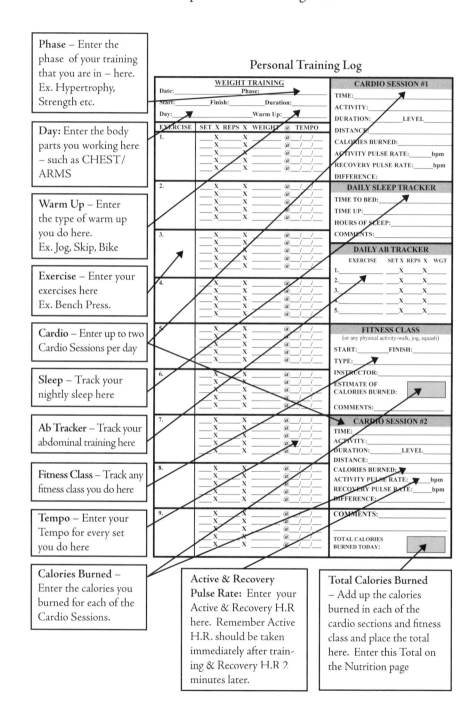

Phase – Enter the phase of your training that you are in – here. Ex. Hypertrophy, Strength etc.

Day: Enter the body parts you working here – such as CHEST/ARMS

Warm Up – Enter the type of warm up you do here. Ex. Jog, Skip, Bike

Exercise – Enter your exercises here Ex. Bench Press.

Cardio – Enter up to two Cardio Sessions per day

Sleep – Track your nightly sleep here

Ab Tracker – Track your abdominal training here

Fitness Class – Track any fitness class you do here

Tempo – Enter your Tempo for every set you do here

Calories Burned – Enter the calories you burned for each of the Cardio Sessions.

Active & Recovery Pulse Rate: Enter your Active & Recovery H.R here. Remember Active H.R. should be taken immediately after training & Recovery H.R 2 minutes later.

Total Calories Burned – Add up the calories burned in each of the cardio sections and fitness class and place the total here. Enter this Total on the Nutrition page

Personal Training Log

WEIGHT TRAINING
Date: _____ Phase: _____
Start: ___ Finish: ___ Duration: ___
Day: _____ Warm Up: _____

EXERCISE	SET X REPS X WEIGHT @ TEMPO
1.	X ___ X ___ @ _/_/_
	X ___ X ___ @ _/_/_
	X ___ X ___ @ _/_/_
	X ___ X ___ @ _/_/_
	X ___ X ___ @ _/_/_
2.	X ___ X ___ @ _/_/_
	X ___ X ___ @ _/_/_
	X ___ X ___ @ _/_/_
	X ___ X ___ @ _/_/_
3.	X ___ X ___ @ _/_/_
	X ___ X ___ @ _/_/_
	X ___ X ___ @ _/_/_
	X ___ X ___ @ _/_/_
4.	X ___ X ___ @ _/_/_
	X ___ X ___ @ _/_/_
	X ___ X ___ @ _/_/_
	X ___ X ___ @ _/_/_
5.	X ___ X ___ @ _/_/_
	X ___ X ___ @ _/_/_
	X ___ X ___ @ _/_/_
	X ___ X ___ @ _/_/_
6.	X ___ X ___ @ _/_/_
	X ___ X ___ @ _/_/_
	X ___ X ___ @ _/_/_
	X ___ X ___ @ _/_/_
7.	X ___ X ___ @ _/_/_
	X ___ X ___ @ _/_/_
	X ___ X ___ @ _/_/_
	X ___ X ___ @ _/_/_
8.	X ___ X ___ @ _/_/_
	X ___ X ___ @ _/_/_
	X ___ X ___ @ _/_/_
	X ___ X ___ @ _/_/_
9.	X ___ X ___ @ _/_/_
	X ___ X ___ @ _/_/_
	X ___ X ___ @ _/_/_
	X ___ X ___ @ _/_/_

CARDIO SESSION #1
TIME: _____
ACTIVITY: _____
DURATION: ___ LEVEL ___
DISTANCE: _____
CALORIES BURNED: _____
ACTIVITY PULSE RATE: ___bpm
RECOVERY PULSE RATE: ___bpm
DIFFERENCE: _____

DAILY SLEEP TRACKER
TIME TO BED: _____
TIME UP: _____
HOURS OF SLEEP: _____
COMMENTS: _____

DAILY AB TRACKER
EXERCISE	SET X REPS X WGT
1.	X ___ X ___
2.	X ___ X ___
3.	X ___ X ___
	X ___ X ___
5.	X ___ X ___

FITNESS CLASS
(or any physical activity-walk, jog, squash)
START: ___ FINISH: ___
TYPE: _____
INSTRUCTOR: _____
ESTIMATE OF CALORIES BURNED: _____
COMMENTS: _____

CARDIO SESSION #2
TIME: _____
ACTIVITY: _____
DURATION: ___ LEVEL ___
DISTANCE: _____
CALORIES BURNED: _____
ACTIVITY PULSE RATE: ___bpm
RECOVERY PULSE RATE: ___bpm
DIFFERENCE: _____

COMMENTS: _____

TOTAL CALORIES BURNED TODAY: _____

Example of Daily Nutrition Tracking

Protein/Fat/Carbs – Track each of these by way of "grams" in each of your meals then add up the totals of each and follow the formula below to determine your total calories for the day. This is a great way to see which type of calories you are consuming.

Meal – Enter your first meal of the day here and so on

Time – Enter the time you eat each meal beside the Meal #.

Points Option – If you are utilizing a "Point" system for the food you consume, simply enter your "Points" for each meal here.

Points Goal – Enter your "Points" goal number at the start of each day here.

Calorie Option – This option allows you to track calories for the food you eat Ex. 2 slices whole wheat bread = 170 calories. Just enter the total calories rather than breaking it down to Protein, Carbs and Fat. This option gives an easy way to track the amount of calories you take in for the day.

Points Total/Difference Enter your "Points" total here and underneath where it says Difference simply subtract your target total at the top from your actual points and put down this number as a plus or minus. Ideally it should say "0".

NUTRITION	Points Goal	CAL *option*	PROT *grams*	FAT *grams*	CARB *grams*
Meal #1 – Time: H₂O_____Cups(L)					
Meal #2 – Time: H₂O_____Cups(L)					
Meal #3 – Time: H₂O_____Cups(L)					
Meal #4 – Time: H₂O_____Cups(L)					
Meal #5 – Time: H₂O_____Cups(L)					
Meal #6 – Time: H₂O_____Cups(L)					
Food Point Total For Today:					
Difference (Goal Points Minus Actual Points)					
Daily Totals: (Add up each nutrient column. Convert each to calories. Add all and enter in "Total Calories".)			g	g	g
Conversion To Calories Multiply Total Grams of Prot X 4 = Calories / Multiply Total Grams of Carb X 4 = Calories / Multiply Total Grams of Fat X 9 = Calories	*Total Calories*		cal	cal	cal
Daily Percentages: (Divide total calories of each nutrient by the Total Number of Calories)			%	%	%
Total Calories Consumed:_____					
VS Difference					
Total Calories Burned:_____					

Total Calories Burned – Add up all the Calories you expended in the day from your weight lifting page and enter it here. Subtract it from Total Calories Consumed for the "Difference"

A Final Note

If you stop and think for a moment about what you have in front of you, you will realize that The Personal Training Log (PTL) is a very powerful tool in helping you to reach your goals.

As a Husband, Father of two daughters, full time Police Officer, part time Personal Trainer, Head Football Coach for Ernestown Secondary School Varsity Football Team, Assistant Strength and Conditioning Coach for the Queen's University Golden Gaels Football Team, a Doping Control Officer for The Canadian Centre For Ethics in Sport, the Head of the Anti-Doping Unit of Neutron Sports a company that promotes Natural Body Building & Fitness Events, I have learned, that due to the type of lives we all lead with various commitments and deadlines, it is sometimes difficult to adhere to a strict nutritional and weight training program.

It is for this reason, I have created the PTL in the manner in which it is presented to you, as a daily system of tracking your workouts and nutrition. I know through personal experience that it may be difficult to get to the gym or eat the right type of foods each day. I to have fallen off the weight training and nutritional wagon, but have always got myself back on. The PTL will help you to get back on or get on for the first time. There is no doubt that it will help you to get organized and focused on attaining your fitness goals!

If you follow the motivational techniques that the PTL offers you and take the time to fill in all the areas, you will have an absolutely incredible history of yourself that you or your personal trainer could evaluate and make recommendations on how you can improve.

The PTL is very simple but POWERFUL! Use it to its fullest potential and you will easily identify where you can make changes to your training, nutrition and lifestyle.

Stay Strong!

Progress Report

Measurements

	Start	Cycle 1 Results	Cycle 2 Results	Cycle 3 Results	Goal	Difference
DATE						
Neck						
Bicep L or R						
Chest						
Waist						
Hips						
Thigh L or R						
Calf L or R						
Weight						
% Body Fat						
Hip/Waist Ratio						

Strength

EXERCISES	Start	Cycle 1 Results	Cycle 2 Results	Cycle 3 Results	Goal	Difference
DATE						
1.						
2.						
3.						
4.						
5.						
6.						
7.						
8.						
9.						
10.						

Notes

Enter Cycle

Personal Fitness Evaluation

1

Date:_____Height:_____Weight:_____Age:_____

Medical History:_____
_____
_____

TESTING:

Resting Heart Rate:_____bpm   Blood Pressure:_____/_____   Body Fat:_____%

Flexibility:_____   Push Ups:_____   Sit Ups:_____   Chin Ups:_____

Other Required Tests & Results:

1._____ [ ]   2._____ [ ]   3._____ [ ]

4._____ [ ]   5._____ [ ]   6._____ [ ]

WAIST TO HIP RATIO:

Waist:_____ Divided by Hips:_____ = [ ]   Women: 0.8 or less
Men: 0.95 or less

GOALS FOR THIS CYCLE:

1._____   3._____

2._____   4._____

YOUR PLAN TO ACHIEVE YOUR GOALS:
Be very specific in your plan, for example you may want to increase your cardio sessions from 20 to 25 minutes or you may want to increase your daily water intake by 1 glass. State this in your plan. Be careful to make your goals REALISTIC and ATTAINABLE. Keep in mind you do not have to use all five spaces provided. Keep it simple!

1._____
2._____
3._____
4._____
5._____

Weight Training Program:

Day 1	Tempo	Day 2	Tempo
1._____	_/_/_	1._____	_/_/_
2._____	_/_/_	2._____	_/_/_
3._____	_/_/_	3._____	_/_/_
4._____	_/_/_	4._____	_/_/_
5._____	_/_/_	5._____	_/_/_
6._____	_/_/_	6._____	_/_/_
7._____	_/_/_	7._____	_/_/_
8._____	_/_/_	8._____	_/_/_
9._____	_/_/_	9._____	_/_/_

Aerobic Exercise Plan:

Type:_____ ___to___ x per week @____ to____min/session

Suggested Training Heart Rate: _____ to_____ beats/min

Aerobic Class Recommendation: _____

Current Eating Habits
(Typical Day)

Breakfast:_____

Snack:_____

Lunch: _____

Snack:_____

Dinner:_____

Evening Snack: _____

Suggested Changes to Eating Habits

Meal 1:_____

Meal 2: _____

Meal 3: _____

Meal 4: _____

Meal 5: _____

Meal 6: _____

Date Photograph taken: _____

Weight: _____ % Body Fat: _____

1

PLACE PHOTO
HERE

Photograph - End of Cycle #1

Date Photograph taken: _____

Weight: _____ % Body Fat: _____

PLACE PHOTO
HERE

Personal Training Log

	WEIGHT TRAINING			CARDIO SESSION #1

WEIGHT TRAINING

Date:_____Phase:_____

Start:_____Finish:_____Duration:_____

Day:_____Warm Up:_____

EXERCISE	SET X REPS X WEIGHT @ TEMPO
1.	___X___X_____@__/__/__
	___X___X_____@__/__/__
	___X___X_____@__/__/__
	___X___X_____@__/__/__
	___X___X_____@__/__/__
2.	___X___X_____@__/__/__
	___X___X_____@__/__/__
	___X___X_____@__/__/__
	___X___X_____@__/__/__
	___X___X_____@__/__/__
3.	___X___X_____@__/__/__
	___X___X_____@__/__/__
	___X___X_____@__/__/__
	___X___X_____@__/__/__
	___X___X_____@__/__/__
4.	___X___X_____@__/__/__
	___X___X_____@__/__/__
	___X___X_____@__/__/__
	___X___X_____@__/__/__
	___X___X_____@__/__/__
5.	___X___X_____@__/__/__
	___X___X_____@__/__/__
	___X___X_____@__/__/__
	___X___X_____@__/__/__
	___X___X_____@__/__/__
6.	___X___X_____@__/__/__
	___X___X_____@__/__/__
	___X___X_____@__/__/__
	___X___X_____@__/__/__
	___X___X_____@__/__/__
7.	___X___X_____@__/__/__
	___X___X_____@__/__/__
	___X___X_____@__/__/__
	___X___X_____@__/__/__
	___X___X_____@__/__/__
8.	___X___X_____@__/__/__
	___X___X_____@__/__/__
	___X___X_____@__/__/__
	___X___X_____@__/__/__
	___X___X_____@__/__/__
9.	___X___X_____@__/__/__
	___X___X_____@__/__/__
	___X___X_____@__/__/__
	___X___X_____@__/__/__
	___X___X_____@__/__/__

CARDIO SESSION #1

TIME:_____

ACTIVITY:_____

DURATION:_____LEVEL_____

DISTANCE:_____

CALORIES BURNED:_____

ACTIVITY PULSE RATE:_____bpm

RECOVERY PULSE RATE:_____bpm

DIFFERENCE:

DAILY SLEEP TRACKER

TIME TO BED:_____

TIME UP:_____

HOURS OF SLEEP:_____

COMMENTS:_____

DAILY AB TRACKER

EXERCISE	SET X REPS X WGT
1._____	___X____X_____
2._____	___X____X_____
3._____	___X____X_____
4._____	___X____X_____
5._____	___X____X_____

FITNESS CLASS

(or any physical activity-walk, jog, squash)

START:_____FINISH:_____

TYPE:_____

INSTRUCTOR:_____

**ESTIMATE OF
CALORIES BURNED:**

COMMENTS:_____

CARDIO SESSION #2

TIME:_____

ACTIVITY:_____

DURATION:_____LEVEL_____

DISTANCE:_____

CALORIES BURNED:_____

ACTIVITY PULSE RATE:_____bpm

RECOVERY PULSE RATE:_____bpm

DIFFERENCE:_____

COMMENTS:_____

**TOTAL CALORIES
BURNED TODAY:**

1

Daily Nutrition Tracking

NUTRITION	Points Goal	CAL *option*	PROT *grams*	FAT *grams*	CARB *grams*
Meal #1 – Time: H₂O____Cups(L)					
Meal #2 – Time: H₂O____Cups(L)					
Meal #3 – Time: H₂O____Cups(L)					
Meal #4 – Time: H₂O____Cups(L)					
Meal #5 – Time: H₂O____Cups(L)					
Meal #6 – Time: H₂O____Cups(L)					

1

Food Point Total For Today:			
Difference (Goal Points Minus Actual Points)			

Daily Totals: *(Add up each nutrient column. Convert each to calories. Add all and enter in "Total Calories")* — g g g

Conversion To Calories
Multiply Total Grams of **Pro X 4** = Calories
Multiply Total Grams of **Carb X 4**=Calories
Multiply Total Grams of **Fat X 9** = Calories

Total Calories — cal cal cal

Daily Percentages: (*Divide total calories of each nutrient by the Total Number of Calories*) — % % %

Total Calories Consumed:_____
VS
Total Calories Burned: _____
Difference

Personal Training Log

WEIGHT TRAINING		CARDIO SESSION #1

WEIGHT TRAINING

Date:_____ Phase:_____

Start:_____ Finish:_____ Duration:_____

Day:_____ Warm Up:_____

EXERCISE	SET X REPS X WEIGHT @ TEMPO
1.	___ X ___ X _____ @__/__/__
	___ X ___ X _____ @__/__/__
	___ X ___ X _____ @__/__/__
	___ X ___ X _____ @__/__/__
	___ X ___ X _____ @__/__/__
2.	___ X ___ X _____ @__/__/__
	___ X ___ X _____ @__/__/__
	___ X ___ X _____ @__/__/__
	___ X ___ X _____ @__/__/__
	___ X ___ X _____ @__/__/__
3.	___ X ___ X _____ @__/__/__
	___ X ___ X _____ @__/__/__
	___ X ___ X _____ @__/__/__
	___ X ___ X _____ @__/__/__
	___ X ___ X _____ @__/__/__
4.	___ X ___ X _____ @__/__/__
	___ X ___ X _____ @__/__/__
	___ X ___ X _____ @__/__/__
	___ X ___ X _____ @__/__/__
	___ X ___ X _____ @__/__/__
5.	___ X ___ X _____ @__/__/__
	___ X ___ X _____ @__/__/__
	___ X ___ X _____ @__/__/__
	___ X ___ X _____ @__/__/__
	___ X ___ X _____ @__/__/__
6.	___ X ___ X _____ @__/__/__
	___ X ___ X _____ @__/__/__
	___ X ___ X _____ @__/__/__
	___ X ___ X _____ @__/__/__
	___ X ___ X _____ @__/__/__
7.	___ X ___ X _____ @__/__/__
	___ X ___ X _____ @__/__/__
	___ X ___ X _____ @__/__/__
	___ X ___ X _____ @__/__/__
	___ X ___ X _____ @__/__/__
8.	___ X ___ X _____ @__/__/__
	___ X ___ X _____ @__/__/__
	___ X ___ X _____ @__/__/__
	___ X ___ X _____ @__/__/__
	___ X ___ X _____ @__/__/__
9.	___ X ___ X _____ @__/__/__
	___ X ___ X _____ @__/__/__
	___ X ___ X _____ @__/__/__
	___ X ___ X _____ @__/__/__
	___ X ___ X _____ @__/__/__

CARDIO SESSION #1

TIME:_____

ACTIVITY:_____

DURATION:_____ LEVEL_____

DISTANCE:_____

CALORIES BURNED:_____

ACTIVITY PULSE RATE:_____bpm

RECOVERY PULSE RATE:_____bpm

DIFFERENCE:

DAILY SLEEP TRACKER

TIME TO BED:_____

TIME UP:_____

HOURS OF SLEEP:_____

COMMENTS:_____

DAILY AB TRACKER

EXERCISE	SET X REPS X WGT
1._____	___ X ___ X _____
2._____	___ X ___ X _____
3._____	___ X ___ X _____
4._____	___ X ___ X _____
5._____	___ X ___ X _____

FITNESS CLASS

(or any physical activity-walk, jog, squash)

START:_____ FINISH:_____

TYPE:_____

INSTRUCTOR:_____

ESTIMATE OF
CALORIES BURNED: [   ]

COMMENTS:_____

CARDIO SESSION #2

TIME:_____

ACTIVITY:_____

DURATION:_____ LEVEL_____

DISTANCE:_____

CALORIES BURNED:_____

ACTIVITY PULSE RATE:_____bpm

RECOVERY PULSE RATE:_____bpm

DIFFERENCE:_____

COMMENTS:_____

_____

TOTAL CALORIES
BURNED TODAY: [   ]

NUTRITION	Points Goal	CAL *option*	PROT *grams*	FAT *grams*	CARB *grams*
Meal #1 – Time: H₂O_____Cups(L)					
Meal #2 – Time: H₂O_____Cups(L)					
Meal #3 – Time: H₂O_____Cups(L)					
Meal #4 – Time: H₂O_____Cups(L)					
Meal #5 – Time: H₂O_____Cups(L)					
Meal #6 – Time: H₂O_____Cups(L)					

	Points Goal		PROT	FAT	CARB
Food Point Total For Today:					
Difference (Goal Points Minus Actual Points)					
Daily Totals: (Add up each nutrient column. Convert each to calories. Add all and enter in "Total Calories")			g	g	g
Conversion To Calories	**Total Calories**				
Multiply Total Grams of **Pro X 4** = Calories					
Multiply Total Grams of **Carb X 4**=Calories			cal	cal	cal
Multiply Total Grams of **Fat X 9** = Calories					
Daily Percentages: (Divide total calories of each nutrient by the Total Number of Calories)			%	%	%

Total Calories Consumed:_____

        VS   *Difference*

Total Calories Burned: _____

Personal Training Log

WEIGHT TRAINING

Date:_____ Phase:_____
Start:_____ Finish:_____ Duration:_____
Day:_____ Warm Up:_____

EXERCISE	SET X REPS X WEIGHT @ TEMPO
1.	___X___X_____@__/__/__
	___X___X_____@__/__/__
	___X___X_____@__/__/__
	___X___X_____@__/__/__
	___X___X_____@__/__/__
2.	___X___X_____@__/__/__
	___X___X_____@__/__/__
	___X___X_____@__/__/__
	___X___X_____@__/__/__
	___X___X_____@__/__/__
3.	___X___X_____@__/__/__
	___X___X_____@__/__/__
	___X___X_____@__/__/__
	___X___X_____@__/__/__
	___X___X_____@__/__/__
4.	___X___X_____@__/__/__
	___X___X_____@__/__/__
	___X___X_____@__/__/__
	___X___X_____@__/__/__
	___X___X_____@__/__/__
5.	___X___X_____@__/__/__
	___X___X_____@__/__/__
	___X___X_____@__/__/__
	___X___X_____@__/__/__
	___X___X_____@__/__/__
6.	___X___X_____@__/__/__
	___X___X_____@__/__/__
	___X___X_____@__/__/__
	___X___X_____@__/__/__
	___X___X_____@__/__/__
7.	___X___X_____@__/__/__
	___X___X_____@__/__/__
	___X___X_____@__/__/__
	___X___X_____@__/__/__
	___X___X_____@__/__/__
8.	___X___X_____@__/__/__
	___X___X_____@__/__/__
	___X___X_____@__/__/__
	___X___X_____@__/__/__
	___X___X_____@__/__/__
9.	___X___X_____@__/__/__
	___X___X_____@__/__/__
	___X___X_____@__/__/__
	___X___X_____@__/__/__
	___X___X_____@__/__/__

CARDIO SESSION #1

TIME:_____
ACTIVITY:_____
DURATION:_____ LEVEL_____
DISTANCE:_____
CALORIES BURNED:_____
ACTIVITY PULSE RATE:_____ bpm
RECOVERY PULSE RATE:_____ bpm
DIFFERENCE:

DAILY SLEEP TRACKER

TIME TO BED:_____
TIME UP:_____
HOURS OF SLEEP:_____
COMMENTS:_____

DAILY AB TRACKER

EXERCISE	SET X REPS X WGT
1._____	___X___X___
2._____	___X___X___
3._____	___X___X___
4._____	___X___X___
5._____	___X___X___

FITNESS CLASS
(or any physical activity-walk, jog, squash)

START:_____ FINISH:_____
TYPE:_____
INSTRUCTOR:_____
ESTIMATE OF CALORIES BURNED: [ ]
COMMENTS:_____

CARDIO SESSION #2

TIME:_____
ACTIVITY:_____
DURATION:_____ LEVEL_____
DISTANCE:_____
CALORIES BURNED:_____
ACTIVITY PULSE RATE:_____ bpm
RECOVERY PULSE RATE:_____ bpm
DIFFERENCE:_____

COMMENTS:_____

TOTAL CALORIES BURNED TODAY: [ ]

Daily Nutrition Tracking

NUTRITION	Points Goal	CAL *option*	PROT *grams*	FAT *grams*	CARB *grams*
Meal #1 – Time: H_2O_____Cups(L)					
Meal #2 – Time: H_2O_____Cups(L)					
Meal #3 – Time: H_2O_____Cups(L)					
Meal #4 – Time: H_2O_____Cups(L)					
Meal #5 – Time: H_2O_____Cups(L)					
Meal #6 – Time: H_2O_____Cups(L)					

Food Point Total For Today:			
Difference (Goal Points Minus Actual Points)			

Daily Totals: (Add up each nutrient column. Convert each to calories. Add all and enter in "Total Calories")   **g   g   g**

Conversion To Calories
Multiply Total Grams of **Pro X 4** = Calories
Multiply Total Grams of **Carb X 4** = Calories
Multiply Total Grams of **Fat X 9** = Calories

Total Calories   **cal   cal   cal**

Daily Percentages: (Divide total calories of each nutrient by the Total Number of Calories)   **%   %   %**

Total Calories Consumed:_____
VS   ***Difference***
Total Calories Burned:_____

Personal Training Log

WEIGHT TRAINING

Date:_____ Phase:_____

Start:_____ Finish:_____ Duration:_____

Day:_____ Warm Up:_____

EXERCISE	SET X REPS X WEIGHT @ TEMPO
1.	____ X ____ X _____ @__/__/__
	____ X ____ X _____ @__/__/__
	____ X ____ X _____ @__/__/__
	____ X ____ X _____ @__/__/__
	____ X ____ X _____ @__/__/__
2.	____ X ____ X _____ @__/__/__
	____ X ____ X _____ @__/__/__
	____ X ____ X _____ @__/__/__
	____ X ____ X _____ @__/__/__
	____ X ____ X _____ @__/__/__
3.	____ X ____ X _____ @__/__/__
	____ X ____ X _____ @__/__/__
	____ X ____ X _____ @__/__/__
	____ X ____ X _____ @__/__/__
	____ X ____ X _____ @__/__/__
4.	____ X ____ X _____ @__/__/__
	____ X ____ X _____ @__/__/__
	____ X ____ X _____ @__/__/__
	____ X ____ X _____ @__/__/__
	____ X ____ X _____ @__/__/__
5.	____ X ____ X _____ @__/__/__
	____ X ____ X _____ @__/__/__
	____ X ____ X _____ @__/__/__
	____ X ____ X _____ @__/__/__
	____ X ____ X _____ @__/__/__
6.	____ X ____ X _____ @__/__/__
	____ X ____ X _____ @__/__/__
	____ X ____ X _____ @__/__/__
	____ X ____ X _____ @__/__/__
	____ X ____ X _____ @__/__/__
7.	____ X ____ X _____ @__/__/__
	____ X ____ X _____ @__/__/__
	____ X ____ X _____ @__/__/__
	____ X ____ X _____ @__/__/__
	____ X ____ X _____ @__/__/__
8.	____ X ____ X _____ @__/__/__
	____ X ____ X _____ @__/__/__
	____ X ____ X _____ @__/__/__
	____ X ____ X _____ @__/__/__
	____ X ____ X _____ @__/__/__
9.	____ X ____ X _____ @__/__/__
	____ X ____ X _____ @__/__/__
	____ X ____ X _____ @__/__/__
	____ X ____ X _____ @__/__/__
	____ X ____ X _____ @__/__/__

CARDIO SESSION #1

TIME:_____

ACTIVITY:_____

DURATION:_____ LEVEL_____

DISTANCE:_____

CALORIES BURNED:_____

ACTIVITY PULSE RATE:_____ bpm

RECOVERY PULSE RATE:_____ bpm

DIFFERENCE:

DAILY SLEEP TRACKER

TIME TO BED:_____

TIME UP:_____

HOURS OF SLEEP:_____

COMMENTS:_____

DAILY AB TRACKER

EXERCISE	SET X REPS X WGT
1._____	____ X ____ X ____
2._____	____ X ____ X ____
3._____	____ X ____ X ____
4._____	____ X ____ X ____
5._____	____ X ____ X ____

FITNESS CLASS

(or any physical activity-walk, jog, squash)

START:_____ FINISH:_____

TYPE:_____

INSTRUCTOR:_____

ESTIMATE OF
CALORIES BURNED: [   ]

COMMENTS:_____

CARDIO SESSION #2

TIME:_____

ACTIVITY:_____

DURATION:_____ LEVEL_____

DISTANCE:_____

CALORIES BURNED:_____

ACTIVITY PULSE RATE:_____ bpm

RECOVERY PULSE RATE:_____ bpm

DIFFERENCE:_____

COMMENTS:_____

_____

TOTAL CALORIES
BURNED TODAY: [   ]

NUTRITION	Points Goal	CAL *option*	PROT *grams*	FAT *grams*	CARB *grams*
Meal #1 – Time: H_2O_____Cups(L)					
Meal #2 – Time: H_2O_____Cups(L)					
Meal #3 – Time: H_2O_____Cups(L)					
Meal #4 – Time: H_2O_____Cups(L)					
Meal #5 – Time: H_2O_____Cups(L)					
Meal #6 – Time: H_2O_____Cups(L)					
Food Point Total For Today:					
Difference (Goal Points Minus Actual Points)					
Daily Totals: (Add up each nutrient column. Convert each to calories. Add all and enter in "Total Calories")			g	g	g
Conversion To Calories Multiply Total Grams of **Pro X 4** = Calories Multiply Total Grams of **Carb X 4**=Calories Multiply Total Grams of **Fat X 9** = Calories	**Total Calories**		cal	cal	cal
Daily Percentages: (Divide total calories of each nutrient by the Total Number of Calories)			%	%	%

Total Calories Consumed:_____

VS   **Difference**

Total Calories Burned: _____

1

Personal Training Log

WEIGHT TRAINING				CARDIO SESSION #1

WEIGHT TRAINING

Date:_____ Phase:_____

Start:_____ Finish:_____ Duration:_____

Day:_____ Warm Up:_____

EXERCISE	SET X REPS X WEIGHT @ TEMPO
1.	___X___X_____@__/__/__
	___X___X_____@__/__/__
	___X___X_____@__/__/__
	___X___X_____@__/__/__
	___X___X_____@__/__/__
2.	___X___X_____@__/__/__
	___X___X_____@__/__/__
	___X___X_____@__/__/__
	___X___X_____@__/__/__
	___X___X_____@__/__/__
3.	___X___X_____@__/__/__
	___X___X_____@__/__/__
	___X___X_____@__/__/__
	___X___X_____@__/__/__
	___X___X_____@__/__/__
4.	___X___X_____@__/__/__
	___X___X_____@__/__/__
	___X___X_____@__/__/__
	___X___X_____@__/__/__
	___X___X_____@__/__/__
5.	___X___X_____@__/__/__
	___X___X_____@__/__/__
	___X___X_____@__/__/__
	___X___X_____@__/__/__
	___X___X_____@__/__/__
6.	___X___X_____@__/__/__
	___X___X_____@__/__/__
	___X___X_____@__/__/__
	___X___X_____@__/__/__
	___X___X_____@__/__/__
7.	___X___X_____@__/__/__
	___X___X_____@__/__/__
	___X___X_____@__/__/__
	___X___X_____@__/__/__
	___X___X_____@__/__/__
8.	___X___X_____@__/__/__
	___X___X_____@__/__/__
	___X___X_____@__/__/__
	___X___X_____@__/__/__
	___X___X_____@__/__/__
9.	___X___X_____@__/__/__
	___X___X_____@__/__/__
	___X___X_____@__/__/__
	___X___X_____@__/__/__
	___X___X_____@__/__/__

CARDIO SESSION #1

TIME:_____

ACTIVITY:_____

DURATION:_____ LEVEL_____

DISTANCE:_____

CALORIES BURNED:_____

ACTIVITY PULSE RATE:_____bpm

RECOVERY PULSE RATE:_____bpm

DIFFERENCE:

DAILY SLEEP TRACKER

TIME TO BED:_____

TIME UP:_____

HOURS OF SLEEP:_____

COMMENTS:_____

DAILY AB TRACKER

EXERCISE	SET X REPS X WGT
1._____	___X___X_____
2._____	___X___X_____
3._____	___X___X_____
4._____	___X___X_____
5._____	___X___X_____

FITNESS CLASS

(or any physical activity-walk, jog, squash)

START:_____ FINISH:_____

TYPE:_____

INSTRUCTOR:_____

ESTIMATE OF
CALORIES BURNED:

COMMENTS:_____

CARDIO SESSION #2

TIME:_____

ACTIVITY:_____

DURATION:_____ LEVEL_____

DISTANCE:_____

CALORIES BURNED:_____

ACTIVITY PULSE RATE:_____bpm

RECOVERY PULSE RATE:_____bpm

DIFFERENCE:

COMMENTS:_____

TOTAL CALORIES
BURNED TODAY:

1

NUTRITION	Points Goal	CAL *option*	PROT *grams*	FAT *grams*	CARB *grams*
Meal #1 – Time: H₂O_____Cups(L)					
Meal #2 – Time: H₂O_____Cups(L)					
Meal #3 – Time: H₂O_____Cups(L)					
Meal #4 – Time: H₂O_____Cups(L)					
Meal #5 – Time: H₂O_____Cups(L)					
Meal #6 Time: H₂O_____Cups(L)					
Food Point Total For Today:					
Difference (Goal Points Minus Actual Points)					
Daily Totals: *(Add up each nutrient column. Convert each to calories. Add all and enter in "Total Calories")*			g	g	g
Conversion To Calories Multiply Total Grams of **Pro X 4** = Calories Multiply Total Grams of **Carb X 4**=Calories Multiply Total Grams of **Fat X 9** = Calories	**Total Calories**		cal	cal	cal
Daily Percentages: *(Divide total calories of each nutrient by the Total Number of Calories)*			___%	___%	___%

Total Calories Consumed:_____

VS   **Difference**

Total Calories Burned: _____

Personal Training Log

EXERCISE	SET X REPS X WEIGHT @ TEMPO
1.	___X___X_____@__/__/__ ___X___X_____@__/__/__ ___X___X_____@__/__/__ ___X___X_____@__/__/__ ___X___X_____@__/__/__
2.	___X___X_____@__/__/__ ___X___X_____@__/__/__ ___X___X_____@__/__/__ ___X___X_____@__/__/__ ___X___X_____@__/__/__
3.	___X___X_____@__/__/__ ___X___X_____@__/__/__ ___X___X_____@__/__/__ ___X___X_____@__/__/__ ___X___X_____@__/__/__
4.	___X___X_____@__/__/__ ___X___X_____@__/__/__ ___X___X_____@__/__/__ ___X___X_____@__/__/__ ___X___X_____@__/__/__
5.	___X___X_____@__/__/__ ___X___X_____@__/__/__ ___X___X_____@__/__/__ ___X___X_____@__/__/__ ___X___X_____@__/__/__
6.	___X___X_____@__/__/__ ___X___X_____@__/__/__ ___X___X_____@__/__/__ ___X___X_____@__/__/__ ___X___X_____@__/__/__
7.	___X___X_____@__/__/__ ___X___X_____@__/__/__ ___X___X_____@__/__/__ ___X___X_____@__/__/__ ___X___X_____@__/__/__
8.	___X___X_____@__/__/__ ___X___X_____@__/__/__ ___X___X_____@__/__/__ ___X___X_____@__/__/__ ___X___X_____@__/__/__
9.	___X___X_____@__/__/__ ___X___X_____@__/__/__ ___X___X_____@__/__/__ ___X___X_____@__/__/__ ___X___X_____@__/__/__

WEIGHT TRAINING

Date:_____ Phase:_____
Start:_____ Finish:_____ Duration:_____
Day:_____ Warm Up:_____

CARDIO SESSION #1

TIME:_____
ACTIVITY:_____
DURATION:_____ LEVEL_____
DISTANCE:_____
CALORIES BURNED:_____
ACTIVITY PULSE RATE:_____bpm
RECOVERY PULSE RATE:_____bpm
DIFFERENCE:_____

DAILY SLEEP TRACKER

TIME TO BED:_____
TIME UP:_____
HOURS OF SLEEP:_____
COMMENTS:_____

DAILY AB TRACKER

EXERCISE	SET X REPS X WGT
1._____	___X___X_____
2._____	___X___X_____
3._____	___X___X_____
4._____	___X___X_____
5._____	___X___X_____

FITNESS CLASS

(or any physical activity-walk, jog, squash)
START:_____ FINISH:_____
TYPE:_____
INSTRUCTOR:_____
ESTIMATE OF
CALORIES BURNED: [____]
COMMENTS:_____

CARDIO SESSION #2

TIME:_____
ACTIVITY:_____
DURATION:_____ LEVEL_____
DISTANCE:_____
CALORIES BURNED:_____
ACTIVITY PULSE RATE:_____bpm
RECOVERY PULSE RATE:_____bpm
DIFFERENCE:_____

COMMENTS:_____

TOTAL CALORIES
BURNED TODAY: [____]

Daily Nutrition Tracking

NUTRITION	Points Goal	CAL *option*	PROT *grams*	FAT *grams*	CARB *grams*
Meal #1 – Time: H₂O____Cups(L)					
Meal #2 – Time: H₂O____Cups(L)					
Meal #3 – Time: H₂O____Cups(L)					
Meal #4 – Time: H₂O____Cups(L)					
Meal #5 – Time: H₂O____Cups(L)					
Meal #6 – Time: H₂O____Cups(L)					
Food Point Total For Today:					
Difference (Goal Points Minus Actual Points)					

Daily Totals: *(Add up each nutrient column. Convert each to calories. Add all and enter in "Total Calories")* — g   g   g

Conversion To Calories
Multiply Total Grams of **Pro X 4** = Calories
Multiply Total Grams of **Carb X 4** = Calories
Multiply Total Grams of **Fat X 9** = Calories

Total Calories — cal   cal   cal

Daily Percentages: *(Divide total calories of each nutrient by the Total Number of Calories)* — %   %   %

Total Calories Consumed:_____
VS   **Difference**
Total Calories Burned: _____

Personal Training Log

1

WEIGHT TRAINING

Date:_____ Phase:_____

Start:_____ Finish:_____ Duration:_____

Day:_____ Warm Up:_____

EXERCISE	SET X REPS X WEIGHT @ TEMPO
1.	___ X ___ X _____ @__ /__ /__ ___ X ___ X _____ @__ /__ /__ ___ X ___ X _____ @__ /__ /__ ___ X ___ X _____ @__ /__ /__ ___ X ___ X _____ @__ /__ /__
2.	___ X ___ X _____ @__ /__ /__ ___ X ___ X _____ @__ /__ /__ ___ X ___ X _____ @__ /__ /__ ___ X ___ X _____ @__ /__ /__ ___ X ___ X _____ @__ /__ /__
3.	___ X ___ X _____ @__ /__ /__ ___ X ___ X _____ @__ /__ /__ ___ X ___ X _____ @__ /__ /__ ___ X ___ X _____ @__ /__ /__ ___ X ___ X _____ @__ /__ /__
4.	___ X ___ X _____ @__ /__ /__ ___ X ___ X _____ @__ /__ /__ ___ X ___ X _____ @__ /__ /__ ___ X ___ X _____ @__ /__ /__ ___ X ___ X _____ @__ /__ /__
5.	___ X ___ X _____ @__ /__ /__ ___ X ___ X _____ @__ /__ /__ ___ X ___ X _____ @__ /__ /__ ___ X ___ X _____ @__ /__ /__ ___ X ___ X _____ @__ /__ /__
6.	___ X ___ X _____ @__ /__ /__ ___ X ___ X _____ @__ /__ /__ ___ X ___ X _____ @__ /__ /__ ___ X ___ X _____ @__ /__ /__ ___ X ___ X _____ @__ /__ /__
7.	___ X ___ X _____ @__ /__ /__ ___ X ___ X _____ @__ /__ /__ ___ X ___ X _____ @__ /__ /__ ___ X ___ X _____ @__ /__ /__ ___ X ___ X _____ @__ /__ /__
8.	___ X ___ X _____ @__ /__ /__ ___ X ___ X _____ @__ /__ /__ ___ X ___ X _____ @__ /__ /__ ___ X ___ X _____ @__ /__ /__ ___ X ___ X _____ @__ /__ /__
9.	___ X ___ X _____ @__ /__ /__ ___ X ___ X _____ @__ /__ /__ ___ X ___ X _____ @__ /__ /__ ___ X ___ X _____ @__ /__ /__ ___ X ___ X _____ @__ /__ /__

CARDIO SESSION #1

TIME:_____

ACTIVITY:_____

DURATION:_____ LEVEL_____

DISTANCE:_____

CALORIES BURNED:_____

ACTIVITY PULSE RATE:_____ bpm

RECOVERY PULSE RATE:_____ bpm

DIFFERENCE:

DAILY SLEEP TRACKER

TIME TO BED:_____

TIME UP:_____

HOURS OF SLEEP:_____

COMMENTS:_____

DAILY AB TRACKER

EXERCISE	SET X REPS X WGT
1._____	___ X ___ X ___
2._____	___ X ___ X ___
3._____	___ X ___ X ___
4._____	___ X ___ X ___
5._____	___ X ___ X ___

FITNESS CLASS

(or any physical activity-walk, jog, squash)

START:_____ FINISH:_____

TYPE:_____

INSTRUCTOR:_____

ESTIMATE OF
CALORIES BURNED: [   ]

COMMENTS:_____

CARDIO SESSION #2

TIME:_____

ACTIVITY:_____

DURATION:_____ LEVEL_____

DISTANCE:_____

CALORIES BURNED:_____

ACTIVITY PULSE RATE:_____ bpm

RECOVERY PULSE RATE:_____ bpm

DIFFERENCE:_____

COMMENTS:_____

TOTAL CALORIES
BURNED TODAY: [   ]

NUTRITION	Points Goal	CAL *option*	PROT *grams*	FAT *grams*	CARB *grams*
Meal #1 – Time:　　　　H₂O____Cups(L)					
Meal #2 – Time:　　　　H₂O____Cups(L)					
Meal #3 – Time:　　　　H₂O____Cups(L)					
Meal #4 – Time:　　　　H₂O____Cups(L)					
Meal #5 – Time:　　　　H₂O____Cups(L)					
Meal #6 – Time:　　　　H₂O____Cups(L)					
Food Point Total For Today:					
Difference (Goal Points Minus Actual Points)					
Daily Totals: (Add up each nutrient column. Convert each to calories. Add all and enter in "Total Calories")			g	g	g
Conversion To Calories Multiply Total Grams of **Pro X 4** = Calories Multiply Total Grams of **Carb X 4**=Calories Multiply Total Grams of **Fat X 9** = Calories	**Total Calories**		cal	cal	cal
Daily Percentages: (Divide total calories of each nutrient by the Total Number of Calories)			%	%	%

Total Calories Consumed: _____
　　　　VS　　　　　　　　　　***Difference***
Total Calories Burned: _____

1

Personal Training Log

WEIGHT TRAINING

Date:_____Phase:_____

Start:_____Finish:_____Duration:_____

Day:_____Warm Up:_____

EXERCISE	SET X REPS X WEIGHT @ TEMPO
1.	___X___X_____@__/__/__ ___X___X_____@__/__/__ ___X___X_____@__/__/__ ___X___X_____@__/__/__ ___X___X_____@__/__/__
2.	___X___X_____@__/__/__ ___X___X_____@__/__/__ ___X___X_____@__/__/__ ___X___X_____@__/__/__ ___X___X_____@__/__/__
3.	___X___X_____@__/__/__ ___X___X_____@__/__/__ ___X___X_____@__/__/__ ___X___X_____@__/__/__ ___X___X_____@__/__/__
4.	___X___X_____@__/__/__ ___X___X_____@__/__/__ ___X___X_____@__/__/__ ___X___X_____@__/__/__ ___X___X_____@__/__/__
5.	___X___X_____@__/__/__ ___X___X_____@__/__/__ ___X___X_____@__/__/__ ___X___X_____@__/__/__ ___X___X_____@__/__/__
6.	___X___X_____@__/__/__ ___X___X_____@__/__/__ ___X___X_____@__/__/__ ___X___X_____@__/__/__ ___X___X_____@__/__/__
7.	___X___X_____@__/__/__ ___X___X_____@__/__/__ ___X___X_____@__/__/__ ___X___X_____@__/__/__ ___X___X_____@__/__/__
8.	___X___X_____@__/__/__ ___X___X_____@__/__/__ ___X___X_____@__/__/__ ___X___X_____@__/__/__ ___X___X_____@__/__/__
9.	___X___X_____@__/__/__ ___X___X_____@__/__/__ ___X___X_____@__/__/__ ___X___X_____@__/__/__ ___X___X_____@__/__/__

CARDIO SESSION #1

TIME:_____

ACTIVITY:_____

DURATION:_____LEVEL_____

DISTANCE:_____

CALORIES BURNED:_____

ACTIVITY PULSE RATE:_____bpm

RECOVERY PULSE RATE:_____bpm

DIFFERENCE:_____

DAILY SLEEP TRACKER

TIME TO BED:_____

TIME UP:_____

HOURS OF SLEEP:_____

COMMENTS:_____

DAILY AB TRACKER

EXERCISE	SET X REPS X WGT
1._____	___X___X_____
2._____	___X___X_____
3._____	___X___X_____
4._____	___X___X_____
5._____	___X___X_____

FITNESS CLASS
(or any physical activity-walk, jog, squash)

START:_____FINISH:_____

TYPE:_____

INSTRUCTOR:_____

ESTIMATE OF
CALORIES BURNED:

COMMENTS:_____

CARDIO SESSION #2

TIME:_____

ACTIVITY:_____

DURATION:_____LEVEL_____

DISTANCE:_____

CALORIES BURNED:_____

ACTIVITY PULSE RATE:_____bpm

RECOVERY PULSE RATE:_____bpm

DIFFERENCE:_____

COMMENTS:_____

TOTAL CALORIES
BURNED TODAY:

1

NUTRITION	Points Goal	CAL *option*	PROT *grams*	FAT *grams*	CARB *grams*
Meal #1 – Time: H_2O____Cups(L)					
Meal #2 – Time: H_2O____Cups(L)					
Meal #3 – Time: H_2O____Cups(L)					
Meal #4 – Time: H_2O____Cups(L)					
Meal #5 – Time: H_2O____Cups(L)					
Meal #6 – Time: H_2O____Cups(L)					
Food Point Total For Today:					
Difference (Goal Points Minus Actual Points)					
Daily Totals: *(Add up each nutrient column. Convert each to calories. Add all and enter in "Total Calories")*			g	g	g
Conversion To Calories *Multiply Total Grams of **Pro** X 4 = Calories* *Multiply Total Grams of **Carb** X 4=Calories* *Multiply Total Grams of **Fat** X 9 = Calories*	***Total Calories***		cal	cal	cal
Daily Percentages: (*Divide total calories of each nutrient by the Total Number of Calories*)			%	%	%

Total Calories Consumed:_____
            VS   ***Difference***
Total Calories Burned: _____

1

Personal Training Log

WEIGHT TRAINING

Date:_____ Phase:_____

Start:_____ Finish:_____ Duration:_____

Day:_____ Warm Up:_____

EXERCISE	SET X REPS X WEIGHT @ TEMPO
1.	___ X ___ X _____ @ __/__/__
	___ X ___ X _____ @ __/__/__
	___ X ___ X _____ @ __/__/__
	___ X ___ X _____ @ __/__/__
	___ X ___ X _____ @ __/__/__
2.	___ X ___ X _____ @ __/__/__
	___ X ___ X _____ @ __/__/__
	___ X ___ X _____ @ __/__/__
	___ X ___ X _____ @ __/__/__
	___ X ___ X _____ @ __/__/__
3.	___ X ___ X _____ @ __/__/__
	___ X ___ X _____ @ __/__/__
	___ X ___ X _____ @ __/__/__
	___ X ___ X _____ @ __/__/__
	___ X ___ X _____ @ __/__/__
4.	___ X ___ X _____ @ __/__/__
	___ X ___ X _____ @ __/__/__
	___ X ___ X _____ @ __/__/__
	___ X ___ X _____ @ __/__/__
	___ X ___ X _____ @ __/__/__
5.	___ X ___ X _____ @ __/__/__
	___ X ___ X _____ @ __/__/__
	___ X ___ X _____ @ __/__/__
	___ X ___ X _____ @ __/__/__
	___ X ___ X _____ @ __/__/__
6.	___ X ___ X _____ @ __/__/__
	___ X ___ X _____ @ __/__/__
	___ X ___ X _____ @ __/__/__
	___ X ___ X _____ @ __/__/__
	___ X ___ X _____ @ __/__/__
7.	___ X ___ X _____ @ __/__/__
	___ X ___ X _____ @ __/__/__
	___ X ___ X _____ @ __/__/__
	___ X ___ X _____ @ __/__/__
	___ X ___ X _____ @ __/__/__
8.	___ X ___ X _____ @ __/__/__
	___ X ___ X _____ @ __/__/__
	___ X ___ X _____ @ __/__/__
	___ X ___ X _____ @ __/__/__
	___ X ___ X _____ @ __/__/__
9.	___ X ___ X _____ @ __/__/__
	___ X ___ X _____ @ __/__/__
	___ X ___ X _____ @ __/__/__
	___ X ___ X _____ @ __/__/__
	___ X ___ X _____ @ __/__/__

CARDIO SESSION #1

TIME:_____

ACTIVITY:_____

DURATION:_____ LEVEL_____

DISTANCE:_____

CALORIES BURNED:_____

ACTIVITY PULSE RATE:_____bpm

RECOVERY PULSE RATE:_____bpm

DIFFERENCE:

DAILY SLEEP TRACKER

TIME TO BED:_____

TIME UP:_____

HOURS OF SLEEP:_____

COMMENTS:_____

DAILY AB TRACKER

EXERCISE	SET X REPS X WGT
1._____	___ X ___ X ___
2._____	___ X ___ X ___
3._____	___ X ___ X ___
4._____	___ X ___ X ___
5._____	___ X ___ X ___

FITNESS CLASS
(or any physical activity-walk, jog, squash)

START:_____ FINISH:_____

TYPE:_____

INSTRUCTOR:_____

ESTIMATE OF
CALORIES BURNED:

COMMENTS:_____

CARDIO SESSION #2

TIME:_____

ACTIVITY:_____

DURATION:_____ LEVEL_____

DISTANCE:_____

CALORIES BURNED:_____

ACTIVITY PULSE RATE:_____bpm

RECOVERY PULSE RATE:_____bpm

DIFFERENCE:_____

COMMENTS:_____

TOTAL CALORIES
BURNED TODAY:

1

Daily Nutrition Tracking

NUTRITION	Points Goal	CAL *option*	PROT *grams*	FAT *grams*	CARB *grams*
Meal #1 – Time: H₂O_____Cups(L)					
Meal #2 – Time: H₂O_____Cups(L)					
Meal #3 – Time: H₂O_____Cups(L)					
Meal #4 – Time: H₂O_____Cups(L)					
Meal #5 – Time: H₂O_____Cups(L)					
Meal #6 – Time: H₂O_____Cups(L)					
Food Point Total For Today:					
Difference (Goal Points Minus Actual Points)					
Daily Totals: *(Add up each nutrient column. Convert each to calories. Add all and enter in "Total Calories")*			g	g	g
Conversion To Calories Multiply Total Grams of **Pro X 4** = Calories / Multiply Total Grams of **Carb X 4**=Calories / Multiply Total Grams of **Fat X 9** = Calories	**Total Calories**		cal	cal	cal
Daily Percentages: (Divide total calories of each nutrient by the Total Number of Calories)			%	%	%

Total Calories Consumed:_____
VS
Total Calories Burned: _____   **Difference**

1

Personal Training Log

WEIGHT TRAINING

Date:_____ Phase:_____

Start:_____ Finish:_____ Duration:_____

Day:_____ Warm Up:_____

EXERCISE	SET X REPS X WEIGHT @ TEMPO
1.	___X___X_____@__/__/__
	___X___X_____@__/__/__
	___X___X_____@__/__/__
	___X___X_____@__/__/__
	___X___X_____@__/__/__
2.	___X___X_____@__/__/__
	___X___X_____@__/__/__
	___X___X_____@__/__/__
	___X___X_____@__/__/__
	___X___X_____@__/__/__
3.	___X___X_____@__/__/__
	___X___X_____@__/__/__
	___X___X_____@__/__/__
	___X___X_____@__/__/__
	___X___X_____@__/__/__
4.	___X___X_____@__/__/__
	___X___X_____@__/__/__
	___X___X_____@__/__/__
	___X___X_____@__/__/__
	___X___X_____@__/__/__
5.	___X___X_____@__/__/__
	___X___X_____@__/__/__
	___X___X_____@__/__/__
	___X___X_____@__/__/__
	___X___X_____@__/__/__
6.	___X___X_____@__/__/__
	___X___X_____@__/__/__
	___X___X_____@__/__/__
	___X___X_____@__/__/__
	___X___X_____@__/__/__
7.	___X___X_____@__/__/__
	___X___X_____@__/__/__
	___X___X_____@__/__/__
	___X___X_____@__/__/__
	___X___X_____@__/__/__
8.	___X___X_____@__/__/__
	___X___X_____@__/__/__
	___X___X_____@__/__/__
	___X___X_____@__/__/__
	___X___X_____@__/__/__
9.	___X___X_____@__/__/__
	___X___X_____@__/__/__
	___X___X_____@__/__/__
	___X___X_____@__/__/__
	___X___X_____@__/__/__

CARDIO SESSION #1

TIME:_____

ACTIVITY:_____

DURATION:_____LEVEL_____

DISTANCE:_____

CALORIES BURNED:_____

ACTIVITY PULSE RATE:_____bpm

RECOVERY PULSE RATE:_____bpm

DIFFERENCE:

DAILY SLEEP TRACKER

TIME TO BED:_____

TIME UP:_____

HOURS OF SLEEP:_____

COMMENTS:_____

DAILY AB TRACKER

EXERCISE	SET X REPS X WGT
1._____	___X___X____
2._____	___X___X____
3._____	___X___X____
4._____	___X___X____
5._____	___X___X____

FITNESS CLASS
(or any physical activity-walk, jog, squash)

START:_____FINISH:_____

TYPE:_____

INSTRUCTOR:_____

ESTIMATE OF
CALORIES BURNED:

COMMENTS:_____

CARDIO SESSION #2

TIME:_____

ACTIVITY:_____

DURATION:_____LEVEL_____

DISTANCE:_____

CALORIES BURNED:_____

ACTIVITY PULSE RATE:_____bpm

RECOVERY PULSE RATE:_____bpm

DIFFERENCE:_____

COMMENTS:_____

TOTAL CALORIES
BURNED TODAY:

1

NUTRITION	Points Goal	CAL *option*	PROT *grams*	FAT *grams*	CARB *grams*
Meal #1 – Time: H$_2$O____Cups(L)					
Meal #2 – Time: H$_2$O____Cups(L)					
Meal #3 – Time: H$_2$O____Cups(L)					
Meal #4 – Time: H$_2$O____Cups(L)					
Meal #5 – Time: H$_2$O____Cups(L)					
Meal #6 – Time: H$_2$O____Cups(L)					
Food Point Total For Today:					
Difference (Goal Points Minus Actual Points)					
Daily Totals: (Add up each nutrient column. Convert each to calories. Add all and enter in "Total Calories")			g	g	g
Conversion To Calories Multiply Total Grams of **Pro X 4** = Calories; Multiply Total Grams of **Carb X 4** = Calories; Multiply Total Grams of **Fat X 9** = Calories	**Total Calories**		cal	cal	cal
Daily Percentages: (Divide total calories of each nutrient by the Total Number of Calories)			___ %	___ %	___ %

Total Calories Consumed:_____
         VS   ***Difference***
Total Calories Burned: _____

Personal Training Log

WEIGHT TRAINING

Date:_____ Phase:_____

Start:_____ Finish:_____ Duration:_____

Day:_____ Warm Up:_____

EXERCISE	SET X REPS X WEIGHT @ TEMPO
1.	___X___X_____@__/__/__
	___X___X_____@__/__/__
	___X___X_____@__/__/__
	___X___X_____@__/__/__
	___X___X_____@__/__/__
2.	___X___X_____@__/__/__
	___X___X_____@__/__/__
	___X___X_____@__/__/__
	___X___X_____@__/__/__
	___X___X_____@__/__/__
3.	___X___X_____@__/__/__
	___X___X_____@__/__/__
	___X___X_____@__/__/__
	___X___X_____@__/__/__
	___X___X_____@__/__/__
4.	___X___X_____@__/__/__
	___X___X_____@__/__/__
	___X___X_____@__/__/__
	___X___X_____@__/__/__
	___X___X_____@__/__/__
5.	___X___X_____@__/__/__
	___X___X_____@__/__/__
	___X___X_____@__/__/__
	___X___X_____@__/__/__
	___X___X_____@__/__/__
6.	___X___X_____@__/__/__
	___X___X_____@__/__/__
	___X___X_____@__/__/__
	___X___X_____@__/__/__
	___X___X_____@__/__/__
7.	___X___X_____@__/__/__
	___X___X_____@__/__/__
	___X___X_____@__/__/__
	___X___X_____@__/__/__
	___X___X_____@__/__/__
8.	___X___X_____@__/__/__
	___X___X_____@__/__/__
	___X___X_____@__/__/__
	___X___X_____@__/__/__
	___X___X_____@__/__/__
9.	___X___X_____@__/__/__
	___X___X_____@__/__/__
	___X___X_____@__/__/__
	___X___X_____@__/__/__
	___X___X_____@__/__/__

CARDIO SESSION #1

TIME:_____

ACTIVITY:_____

DURATION:_____ LEVEL_____

DISTANCE:_____

CALORIES BURNED:_____

ACTIVITY PULSE RATE:_____bpm

RECOVERY PULSE RATE:_____bpm

DIFFERENCE:_____

DAILY SLEEP TRACKER

TIME TO BED:_____

TIME UP:_____

HOURS OF SLEEP:_____

COMMENTS:_____

DAILY AB TRACKER

EXERCISE	SET X REPS X WGT
1._____	___X___X_____
2._____	___X___X_____
3._____	___X___X_____
4._____	___X___X_____
5._____	___X___X_____

FITNESS CLASS

(or any physical activity-walk, jog, squash)

START:_____ FINISH:_____

TYPE:_____

INSTRUCTOR:_____

ESTIMATE OF
CALORIES BURNED:

COMMENTS:_____

CARDIO SESSION #2

TIME:_____

ACTIVITY:_____

DURATION:_____ LEVEL_____

DISTANCE:_____

CALORIES BURNED:_____

ACTIVITY PULSE RATE:_____bpm

RECOVERY PULSE RATE:_____bpm

DIFFERENCE:_____

COMMENTS:_____

TOTAL CALORIES
BURNED TODAY:

Daily Nutrition Tracking

NUTRITION	Points Goal	CAL *option*	PROT *grams*	FAT *grams*	CARB *grams*
Meal #1 – Time:　　　H$_2$O____Cups(L)					
Meal #2 – Time:　　　H$_2$O____Cups(L)					
Meal #3 – Time:　　　H$_2$O____Cups(L)					
Meal #4 – Time:　　　H$_2$O____Cups(L)					
Meal #5 – Time:　　　H$_2$O____Cups(L)					
Meal #6 – Time:　　　H$_2$O____Cups(L)					
Food Point Total For Today:					
Difference (Goal Points Minus Actual Points)					

Daily Totals: *(Add up each nutrient column. Convert each to calories. Add all and enter in "Total Calories")*　　g　g　g

Conversion To Calories
Multiply Total Grams of **Pro X 4** = Calories
Multiply Total Grams of **Carb X 4**=Calories
Multiply Total Grams of **Fat X 9** = Calories

Total Calories　　cal　cal　cal

Daily Percentages: (Divide total calories of each nutrient by the Total Number of Calories)　　%　%　%

Total Calories Consumed:_____
VS　　　**Difference**
Total Calories Burned: _____

Personal Training Log

1

WEIGHT TRAINING

Date:_____ Phase:_____

Start:_____ Finish:_____ Duration:_____

Day:_____ Warm Up:_____

EXERCISE	SET X REPS X WEIGHT @ TEMPO
1.	___X___X_____@__/__/__
	___X___X_____@__/__/__
	___X___X_____@__/__/__
	___X___X_____@__/__/__
	___X___X_____@__/__/__
2.	___X___X_____@__/__/__
	___X___X_____@__/__/__
	___X___X_____@__/__/__
	___X___X_____@__/__/__
	___X___X_____@__/__/__
3.	___X___X_____@__/__/__
	___X___X_____@__/__/__
	___X___X_____@__/__/__
	___X___X_____@__/__/__
	___X___X_____@__/__/__
4.	___X___X_____@__/__/__
	___X___X_____@__/__/__
	___X___X_____@__/__/__
	___X___X_____@__/__/__
	___X___X_____@__/__/__
5.	___X___X_____@__/__/__
	___X___X_____@__/__/__
	___X___X_____@__/__/__
	___X___X_____@__/__/__
	___X___X_____@__/__/__
6.	___X___X_____@__/__/__
	___X___X_____@__/__/__
	___X___X_____@__/__/__
	___X___X_____@__/__/__
	___X___X_____@__/__/__
7.	___X___X_____@__/__/__
	___X___X_____@__/__/__
	___X___X_____@__/__/__
	___X___X_____@__/__/__
	___X___X_____@__/__/__
8.	___X___X_____@__/__/__
	___X___X_____@__/__/__
	___X___X_____@__/__/__
	___X___X_____@__/__/__
	___X___X_____@__/__/__
9.	___X___X_____@__/__/__
	___X___X_____@__/__/__
	___X___X_____@__/__/__
	___X___X_____@__/__/__
	___X___X_____@__/__/__

CARDIO SESSION #1

TIME:_____

ACTIVITY:_____

DURATION:_____LEVEL_____

DISTANCE:_____

CALORIES BURNED:_____

ACTIVITY PULSE RATE:_____bpm

RECOVERY PULSE RATE:_____bpm

DIFFERENCE:

DAILY SLEEP TRACKER

TIME TO BED:_____

TIME UP:_____

HOURS OF SLEEP:_____

COMMENTS:_____

DAILY AB TRACKER

EXERCISE	SET X REPS X WGT
1._____	___X___X___
2._____	___X___X___
3._____	___X___X___
4._____	___X___X___
5._____	___X___X___

FITNESS CLASS

(or any physical activity-walk, jog, squash)

START:_____FINISH:_____

TYPE:_____

INSTRUCTOR:_____

ESTIMATE OF
CALORIES BURNED:

CARDIO SESSION #2

TIME:_____

ACTIVITY:_____

DURATION:_____LEVEL_____

DISTANCE:_____

CALORIES BURNED:_____

ACTIVITY PULSE RATE:_____bpm

RECOVERY PULSE RATE:_____bpm

DIFFERENCE:

COMMENTS:_____

TOTAL CALORIES
BURNED TODAY:

Daily Nutrition Tracking

NUTRITION	Points Goal	CAL *option*	PROT *grams*	FAT *grams*	CARB *grams*
Meal #1 – Time: H₂O____Cups(L)					
Meal #2 – Time: H₂O____Cups(L)					
Meal #3 – Time: H₂O____Cups(L)					
Meal #4 – Time: H₂O____Cups(L)					
Meal #5 – Time: H₂O____Cups(L)					
Meal #6 Time: H₂O____Cups(L)					

Food Point Total For Today:	
Difference (Goal Points Minus Actual Points)	

Daily Totals: *(Add up each nutrient column. Convert each to calories. Add all and enter in "Total Calories")*   g   g   g

Conversion To Calories Multiply Total Grams of **Pro X 4** = Calories Multiply Total Grams of **Carb X 4**=Calories Multiply Total Grams of **Fat X 9** = Calories	**Total Calories**	cal	cal	cal

Daily Percentages: *(Divide total calories of each nutrient by the Total Number of Calories)*   ___ %   ___ %   ___ %

Total Calories Consumed:_____
VS   **Difference**
Total Calories Burned: _____

Personal Training Log

	WEIGHT TRAINING				CARDIO SESSION #1

WEIGHT TRAINING

Date:_____ Phase:_____

Start:_____ Finish:_____ Duration:_____

Day:_____ Warm Up:_____

EXERCISE	SET X REPS X WEIGHT @ TEMPO
1.	___ X ___ X _____ @ __/__/__
	___ X ___ X _____ @ __/__/__
	___ X ___ X _____ @ __/__/__
	___ X ___ X _____ @ __/__/__
	___ X ___ X _____ @ __/__/__
2.	___ X ___ X _____ @ __/__/__
	___ X ___ X _____ @ __/__/__
	___ X ___ X _____ @ __/__/__
	___ X ___ X _____ @ __/__/__
	___ X ___ X _____ @ __/__/__
3.	___ X ___ X _____ @ __/__/__
	___ X ___ X _____ @ __/__/__
	___ X ___ X _____ @ __/__/__
	___ X ___ X _____ @ __/__/__
	___ X ___ X _____ @ __/__/__
4.	___ X ___ X _____ @ __/__/__
	___ X ___ X _____ @ __/__/__
	___ X ___ X _____ @ __/__/__
	___ X ___ X _____ @ __/__/__
	___ X ___ X _____ @ __/__/__
5.	___ X ___ X _____ @ __/__/__
	___ X ___ X _____ @ __/__/__
	___ X ___ X _____ @ __/__/__
	___ X ___ X _____ @ __/__/__
	___ X ___ X _____ @ __/__/__
6.	___ X ___ X _____ @ __/__/__
	___ X ___ X _____ @ __/__/__
	___ X ___ X _____ @ __/__/__
	___ X ___ X _____ @ __/__/__
	___ X ___ X _____ @ __/__/__
7.	___ X ___ X _____ @ __/__/__
	___ X ___ X _____ @ __/__/__
	___ X ___ X _____ @ __/__/__
	___ X ___ X _____ @ __/__/__
	___ X ___ X _____ @ __/__/__
8.	___ X ___ X _____ @ __/__/__
	___ X ___ X _____ @ __/__/__
	___ X ___ X _____ @ __/__/__
	___ X ___ X _____ @ __/__/__
	___ X ___ X _____ @ __/__/__
9.	___ X ___ X _____ @ __/__/__
	___ X ___ X _____ @ __/__/__
	___ X ___ X _____ @ __/__/__
	___ X ___ X _____ @ __/__/__
	___ X ___ X _____ @ __/__/__

CARDIO SESSION #1

TIME:_____

ACTIVITY:_____

DURATION:_____ LEVEL_____

DISTANCE:_____

CALORIES BURNED:_____

ACTIVITY PULSE RATE:_____ bpm

RECOVERY PULSE RATE:_____ bpm

DIFFERENCE:

DAILY SLEEP TRACKER

TIME TO BED:_____

TIME UP:_____

HOURS OF SLEEP:_____

COMMENTS:_____

DAILY AB TRACKER

EXERCISE	SET X REPS X WGT
1._____	___ X ___ X _____
2._____	___ X ___ X _____
3._____	___ X ___ X _____
4._____	___ X ___ X _____
5._____	___ X ___ X _____

FITNESS CLASS

(or any physical activity-walk, jog, squash)

START:_____ FINISH:_____

TYPE:_____

INSTRUCTOR:_____

ESTIMATE OF
CALORIES BURNED:

COMMENTS:_____

CARDIO SESSION #2

TIME:_____

ACTIVITY:_____

DURATION:_____ LEVEL_____

DISTANCE:_____

CALORIES BURNED:_____

ACTIVITY PULSE RATE:_____ bpm

RECOVERY PULSE RATE:_____ bpm

DIFFERENCE:_____

COMMENTS:_____

TOTAL CALORIES
BURNED TODAY:

NUTRITION	Points Goal	CAL *option*	PROT *grams*	FAT *grams*	CARB *grams*
Meal #1 – Time: H₂O____Cups(L)					
Meal #2 – Time: H₂O____Cups(L)					
Meal #3 – Time: H₂O____Cups(L)					
Meal #4 – Time: H₂O____Cups(L)					
Meal #5 – Time: H₂O____Cups(L)					
Meal #6 Time: H₂O____Cups(L)					

Food Point Total For Today:				
Difference *(Goal Points Minus Actual Points)*				
Daily Totals: *(Add up each nutrient column. Convert each to calories. Add all and enter in "Total Calories")*		*g*	*g*	*g*

Conversion To Calories
Multiply Total Grams of **Pro X 4** = Calories
Multiply Total Grams of **Carb X 4** = Calories
Multiply Total Grams of **Fat X 9** = Calories

Total Calories		*cal*	*cal*	*cal*

Daily Percentages: *(Divide total calories of each nutrient by the Total Number of Calories)*

	%	*%*	*%*

Total Calories Consumed:_____
         VS   **Difference**
Total Calories Burned: _____

1

Personal Training Log

WEIGHT TRAINING

Date:_____ Phase:_____

Start:_____ Finish:_____ Duration:_____

Day:_____ Warm Up:_____

EXERCISE	SET X REPS X WEIGHT @ TEMPO
1.	___X___X_____@__/__/__
	___X___X_____@__/__/__
	___X___X_____@__/__/__
	___X___X_____@__/__/__
	___X___X_____@__/__/__
2.	___X___X_____@__/__/__
	___X___X_____@__/__/__
	___X___X_____@__/__/__
	___X___X_____@__/__/__
	___X___X_____@__/__/__
3.	___X___X_____@__/__/__
	___X___X_____@__/__/__
	___X___X_____@__/__/__
	___X___X_____@__/__/__
	___X___X_____@__/__/__
4.	___X___X_____@__/__/__
	___X___X_____@__/__/__
	___X___X_____@__/__/__
	___X___X_____@__/__/__
	___X___X_____@__/__/__
5.	___X___X_____@__/__/__
	___X___X_____@__/__/__
	___X___X_____@__/__/__
	___X___X_____@__/__/__
	___X___X_____@__/__/__
6.	___X___X_____@__/__/__
	___X___X_____@__/__/__
	___X___X_____@__/__/__
	___X___X_____@__/__/__
	___X___X_____@__/__/__
7.	___X___X_____@__/__/__
	___X___X_____@__/__/__
	___X___X_____@__/__/__
	___X___X_____@__/__/__
	___X___X_____@__/__/__
8.	___X___X_____@__/__/__
	___X___X_____@__/__/__
	___X___X_____@__/__/__
	___X___X_____@__/__/__
	___X___X_____@__/__/__
9.	___X___X_____@__/__/__
	___X___X_____@__/__/__
	___X___X_____@__/__/__
	___X___X_____@__/__/__
	___X___X_____@__/__/__

1

CARDIO SESSION #1

TIME:_____

ACTIVITY:_____

DURATION:_____LEVEL_____

DISTANCE:_____

CALORIES BURNED:_____

ACTIVITY PULSE RATE:_____bpm

RECOVERY PULSE RATE:_____bpm

DIFFERENCE:

DAILY SLEEP TRACKER

TIME TO BED:_____

TIME UP:_____

HOURS OF SLEEP:_____

COMMENTS:_____

DAILY AB TRACKER

EXERCISE	SET X REPS X WGT
1._____	___X___X_____
2._____	___X___X_____
3._____	___X___X_____
4._____	___X___X_____
5._____	___X___X_____

FITNESS CLASS
(or any physical activity-walk, jog, squash)

START:_____FINISH:_____

TYPE:_____

INSTRUCTOR:_____

ESTIMATE OF
CALORIES BURNED:

COMMENTS:_____

CARDIO SESSION #2

TIME:_____

ACTIVITY:_____

DURATION:_____LEVEL_____

DISTANCE:_____

CALORIES BURNED:_____

ACTIVITY PULSE RATE:_____bpm

RECOVERY PULSE RATE:_____bpm

DIFFERENCE:_____

COMMENTS:_____

TOTAL CALORIES
BURNED TODAY:

Daily Nutrition Tracking

NUTRITION	Points Goal	CAL option	PROT grams	FAT grams	CARB grams
Meal #1 – Time: H₂O_____Cups(L)					
Meal #2 – Time: H₂O_____Cups(L)					
Meal #3 – Time: H₂O_____Cups(L)					
Meal #4 – Time: H₂O_____Cups(L)					
Meal #5 – Time: H₂O_____Cups(L)					
Meal #6 – Time: H₂O_____Cups(L)					
Food Point Total For Today:					
Difference (Goal Points Minus Actual Points)					

Daily Totals: *(Add up each nutrient column. Convert each to calories. Add all and enter in "Total Calories")* — g g g

Conversion To Calories
Multiply Total Grams of **Pro X 4** = Calories
Multiply Total Grams of **Carb X 4** =Calories
Multiply Total Grams of **Fat X 9** − Calories

Total Calories — cal cal cal

Daily Percentages: *(Divide total calories of each nutrient by the Total Number of Calories)* — % % %

Total Calories Consumed:_____
VS   **Difference**
Total Calories Burned: _____

1

Personal Training Log

WEIGHT TRAINING

Date:_____ Phase:_____

Start:_____ Finish:_____ Duration:_____

Day:_____ Warm Up:_____

EXERCISE	SET X REPS X WEIGHT @ TEMPO
1.	___ X ___ X _____ @__/__/__
	___ X ___ X _____ @__/__/__
	___ X ___ X _____ @__/__/__
	___ X ___ X _____ @__/__/__
	___ X ___ X _____ @__/__/__
2.	___ X ___ X _____ @__/__/__
	___ X ___ X _____ @__/__/__
	___ X ___ X _____ @__/__/__
	___ X ___ X _____ @__/__/__
	___ X ___ X _____ @__/__/__
3.	___ X ___ X _____ @__/__/__
	___ X ___ X _____ @__/__/__
	___ X ___ X _____ @__/__/__
	___ X ___ X _____ @__/__/__
	___ X ___ X _____ @__/__/__
4.	___ X ___ X _____ @__/__/__
	___ X ___ X _____ @__/__/__
	___ X ___ X _____ @__/__/__
	___ X ___ X _____ @__/__/__
	___ X ___ X _____ @__/__/__
5.	___ X ___ X _____ @__/__/__
	___ X ___ X _____ @__/__/__
	___ X ___ X _____ @__/__/__
	___ X ___ X _____ @__/__/__
	___ X ___ X _____ @__/__/__
6.	___ X ___ X _____ @__/__/__
	___ X ___ X _____ @__/__/__
	___ X ___ X _____ @__/__/__
	___ X ___ X _____ @__/__/__
	___ X ___ X _____ @__/__/__
7.	___ X ___ X _____ @__/__/__
	___ X ___ X _____ @__/__/__
	___ X ___ X _____ @__/__/__
	___ X ___ X _____ @__/__/__
	___ X ___ X _____ @__/__/__
8.	___ X ___ X _____ @__/__/__
	___ X ___ X _____ @__/__/__
	___ X ___ X _____ @__/__/__
	___ X ___ X _____ @__/__/__
	___ X ___ X _____ @__/__/__
9.	___ X ___ X _____ @__/__/__
	___ X ___ X _____ @__/__/__
	___ X ___ X _____ @__/__/__
	___ X ___ X _____ @__/__/__
	___ X ___ X _____ @__/__/__

CARDIO SESSION #1

TIME:_____

ACTIVITY:_____

DURATION:_____ LEVEL_____

DISTANCE:_____

CALORIES BURNED:_____

ACTIVITY PULSE RATE:_____bpm

RECOVERY PULSE RATE:_____bpm

DIFFERENCE:

DAILY SLEEP TRACKER

TIME TO BED:_____

TIME UP:_____

HOURS OF SLEEP:_____

COMMENTS:_____

DAILY AB TRACKER

EXERCISE	SET X REPS X WGT
1._____	___ X ___ X ___
2._____	___ X ___ X ___
3._____	___ X ___ X ___
4._____	___ X ___ X ___
5._____	___ X ___ X ___

FITNESS CLASS
(or any physical activity-walk, jog, squash)

START:_____ FINISH:_____

TYPE:_____

INSTRUCTOR:_____

ESTIMATE OF
CALORIES BURNED: [   ]

COMMENTS:_____

CARDIO SESSION #2

TIME:_____

ACTIVITY:_____

DURATION:_____ LEVEL_____

DISTANCE:_____

CALORIES BURNED:_____

ACTIVITY PULSE RATE:_____bpm

RECOVERY PULSE RATE:_____bpm

DIFFERENCE:_____

COMMENTS:_____

TOTAL CALORIES
BURNED TODAY: [   ]

1

NUTRITION	Points Goal	CAL *option*	PROT *grams*	FAT *grams*	CARB *grams*
Meal #1 – Time: H$_2$O_____Cups(L)					
Meal #2 – Time: H$_2$O_____Cups(L)					
Meal #3 – Time: H$_2$O_____Cups(L)					
Meal #4 – Time: H$_2$O_____Cups(L)					
Meal #5 – Time: H$_2$O_____Cups(L)					
Meal #6 – Time: H$_2$O_____Cups(L)					

1

Food Point Total For Today:		
Difference (Goal Points Minus Actual Points)		

Daily Totals: *(Add up each nutrient column. Convert each to calories. Add all and enter in "Total Calories")*   g   g   g

Conversion To Calories *Multiply Total Grams of **Pro X 4** = Calories* *Multiply Total Grams of **Carb X 4**=Calories* *Multiply Total Grams of **Fat X 9** = Calories*	**Total Calories**	cal	cal	cal

Daily Percentages: *(Divide total calories of each nutrient by the Total Number of Calories)*   ___%   ___%   ___%

Total Calories Consumed:_____
                VS   **Difference**
Total Calories Burned: _____

Personal Training Log

<table>
<tr><td colspan="2">

WEIGHT TRAINING

Date:_____Phase:_____

Start:_____Finish:_____Duration:_____

Day:_____Warm Up:_____

</td><td colspan="2">

CARDIO SESSION #1

TIME:_____

ACTIVITY:_____

DURATION:_____LEVEL_____

DISTANCE:_____

CALORIES BURNED:_____

ACTIVITY PULSE RATE:_____bpm

RECOVERY PULSE RATE:_____bpm

DIFFERENCE:

</td></tr>
</table>

EXERCISE	SET X REPS X WEIGHT @ TEMPO
1.	___X___X _____ @__/__/__
	___X___X _____ @__/__/__
	___X___X _____ @__/__/__
	___X___X _____ @__/__/__
	___X___X _____ @__/__/__

DAILY SLEEP TRACKER

2.	___X___X _____ @__/__/__
	___X___X _____ @__/__/__
	___X___X _____ @__/__/__
	___X___X _____ @__/__/__
	___X___X _____ @__/__/__

TIME TO BED:_____

TIME UP:_____

HOURS OF SLEEP:_____

3.	___X___X _____ @__/__/__
	___X___X _____ @__/__/__
	___X___X _____ @__/__/__
	___X___X _____ @__/__/__
	___X___X _____ @__/__/__

COMMENTS:_____

DAILY AB TRACKER

	EXERCISE	SET X REPS X WGT
1.	_____	___X___X____
2.	_____	___X___X____
3.	_____	___X___X____
4.	_____	___X___X____
5.	_____	___X___X____

4.	___X___X _____ @__/__/__
	___X___X _____ @__/__/__
	___X___X _____ @__/__/__
	___X___X _____ @__/__/__
	___X___X _____ @__/__/__

FITNESS CLASS
(or any physical activity-walk, jog, squash)

5.	___X___X _____ @__/__/__
	___X___X _____ @__/__/__
	___X___X _____ @__/__/__
	___X___X _____ @__/__/__
	___X___X _____ @__/__/__

START:_____FINISH:_____

TYPE:_____

6.	___X___X _____ @__/__/__
	___X___X _____ @__/__/__
	___X___X _____ @__/__/__
	___X___X _____ @__/__/__
	___X___X _____ @__/__/__

INSTRUCTOR:_____

ESTIMATE OF
CALORIES BURNED:

COMMENTS:_____

7.	___X___X _____ @__/__/__
	___X___X _____ @__/__/__
	___X___X _____ @__/__/__
	___X___X _____ @__/__/__
	___X___X _____ @__/__/__

CARDIO SESSION #2

TIME:_____

ACTIVITY:_____

DURATION:_____LEVEL_____

DISTANCE:_____

8.	___X___X _____ @__/__/__
	___X___X _____ @__/__/__
	___X___X _____ @__/__/__
	___X___X _____ @__/__/__
	___X___X _____ @__/__/__

CALORIES BURNED:_____

ACTIVITY PULSE RATE:_____bpm

RECOVERY PULSE RATE:_____bpm

DIFFERENCE: _____

9.	___X___X _____ @__/__/__
	___X___X _____ @__/__/__
	___X___X _____ @__/__/__
	___X___X _____ @__/__/__
	___X___X _____ @__/__/__

COMMENTS:_____

TOTAL CALORIES
BURNED TODAY:

1

Daily Nutrition Tracking

NUTRITION	Points Goal	CAL *option*	PROT *grams*	FAT *grams*	CARB *grams*
Meal #1 – Time: H₂O____Cups(L)					
Meal #2 – Time: H₂O____Cups(L)					
Meal #3 – Time: H₂O____Cups(L)					
Meal #4 – Time: H₂O____Cups(L)					
Meal #5 – Time: H₂O____Cups(L)					
Meal #6 – Time: H₂O____Cups(L)					

Food Point Total For Today:

Difference (Goal Points Minus Actual Points)

Daily Totals: (Add up each nutrient column. Convert each to calories. Add all and enter in "Total Calories")   g   g   g

Conversion To Calories
Multiply Total Grams of **Pro X 4** = Calories
Multiply Total Grams of **Carb X 4** = Calories
Multiply Total Grams of **Fat X 9** = Calories

Total Calories   cal   cal   cal

Daily Percentages: (Divide total calories of each nutrient by the Total Number of Calories)   %   %   %

Total Calories Consumed:_____

VS   *Difference*

Total Calories Burned:_____

Personal Training Log

WEIGHT TRAINING

Date:_____ Phase:_____

Start:_____ Finish:_____ Duration:_____

Day:_____ Warm Up:_____

EXERCISE	SET X REPS X WEIGHT @ TEMPO
1.	___X___X____ @__/__/__
	___X___X____ @__/__/__
	___X___X____ @__/__/__
	___X___X____ @__/__/__
	___X___X____ @__/__/__
2.	___X___X____ @__/__/__
	___X___X____ @__/__/__
	___X___X____ @__/__/__
	___X___X____ @__/__/__
	___X___X____ @__/__/__
3.	___X___X____ @__/__/__
	___X___X____ @__/__/__
	___X___X____ @__/__/__
	___X___X____ @__/__/__
	___X___X____ @__/__/__
4.	___X___X____ @__/__/__
	___X___X____ @__/__/__
	___X___X____ @__/__/__
	___X___X____ @__/__/__
	___X___X____ @__/__/__
5.	___X___X____ @__/__/__
	___X___X____ @__/__/__
	___X___X____ @__/__/__
	___X___X____ @__/__/__
	___X___X____ @__/__/__
6.	___X___X____ @__/__/__
	___X___X____ @__/__/__
	___X___X____ @__/__/__
	___X___X____ @__/__/__
	___X___X____ @__/__/__
7.	___X___X____ @__/__/__
	___X___X____ @__/__/__
	___X___X____ @__/__/__
	___X___X____ @__/__/__
	___X___X____ @__/__/__
8.	___X___X____ @__/__/__
	___X___X____ @__/__/__
	___X___X____ @__/__/__
	___X___X____ @__/__/__
	___X___X____ @__/__/__
9.	___X___X____ @__/__/__
	___X___X____ @__/__/__
	___X___X____ @__/__/__
	___X___X____ @__/__/__
	___X___X____ @__/__/__

CARDIO SESSION #1

TIME:_____

ACTIVITY:_____

DURATION:_____ LEVEL_____

DISTANCE:_____

CALORIES BURNED:_____

ACTIVITY PULSE RATE:_____bpm

RECOVERY PULSE RATE:_____bpm

DIFFERENCE:

DAILY SLEEP TRACKER

TIME TO BED:_____

TIME UP:_____

HOURS OF SLEEP:_____

COMMENTS:_____

DAILY AB TRACKER

EXERCISE	SET X REPS X WGT
1._____	___X___X____
2._____	___X___X____
3._____	___X___X____
4._____	___X___X____
5._____	___X___X____

FITNESS CLASS
(or any physical activity-walk, jog, squash)

START:_____ FINISH:_____

TYPE:_____

INSTRUCTOR:_____

ESTIMATE OF
CALORIES BURNED:

COMMENTS:_____

CARDIO SESSION #2

TIME:_____

ACTIVITY:_____

DURATION:_____ LEVEL_____

DISTANCE:_____

CALORIES BURNED:_____

ACTIVITY PULSE RATE:_____bpm

RECOVERY PULSE RATE:_____bpm

DIFFERENCE:_____

COMMENTS:

TOTAL CALORIES
BURNED TODAY:

Daily Nutrition Tracking

NUTRITION	Points Goal	CAL *option*	PROT *grams*	FAT *grams*	CARB *grams*
Meal #1 – Time: H₂O_____Cups(L)					
Meal #2 – Time: H₂O_____Cups(L)					
Meal #3 – Time: H₂O_____Cups(L)					
Meal #4 – Time: H₂O_____Cups(L)					
Meal #5 – Time: H₂O_____Cups(L)					
Meal #6 – Time: H₂O Cups(L)					

Food Point Total For Today:		
Difference (Goal Points Minus Actual Points)		

Daily Totals: *(Add up each nutrient column. Convert each to calories. Add all and enter in "Total Calories")* — g | g | g

Conversion To Calories
Multiply Total Grams of **Pro X 4** = Calories
Multiply Total Grams of **Carb X 4**=Calories
Multiply Total Grams of **Fat X 9** = Calories

Total Calories — cal | cal | cal

Daily Percentages: (*Divide total calories of each nutrient by the Total Number of Calories*) — % | % | %

Total Calories Consumed:_____
VS   **Difference**
Total Calories Burned: _____

Personal Training Log

WEIGHT TRAINING

Date:_____ Phase:_____

Start:_____ Finish:_____ Duration:_____

Day:_____ Warm Up:_____

EXERCISE	SET X REPS X WEIGHT @ TEMPO
1.	___X___X___@__/__/__ ___X___X___@__/__/__ ___X___X___@__/__/__ ___X___X___@__/__/__ ___X___X___@__/__/__
2.	___X___X___@__/__/__ ___X___X___@__/__/__ ___X___X___@__/__/__ ___X___X___@__/__/__ ___X___X___@__/__/__
3.	___X___X___@__/__/__ ___X___X___@__/__/__ ___X___X___@__/__/__ ___X___X___@__/__/__ ___X___X___@__/__/__
4.	___X___X___@__/__/__ ___X___X___@__/__/__ ___X___X___@__/__/__ ___X___X___@__/__/__ ___X___X___@__/__/__
5.	___X___X___@__/__/__ ___X___X___@__/__/__ ___X___X___@__/__/__ ___X___X___@__/__/__ ___X___X___@__/__/__
6.	___X___X___@__/__/__ ___X___X___@__/__/__ ___X___X___@__/__/__ ___X___X___@__/__/__ ___X___X___@__/__/__
7.	___X___X___@__/__/__ ___X___X___@__/__/__ ___X___X___@__/__/__ ___X___X___@__/__/__ ___X___X___@__/__/__
8.	___X___X___@__/__/__ ___X___X___@__/__/__ ___X___X___@__/__/__ ___X___X___@__/__/__ ___X___X___@__/__/__
9.	___X___X___@__/__/__ ___X___X___@__/__/__ ___X___X___@__/__/__ ___X___X___@__/__/__ ___X___X___@__/__/__

CARDIO SESSION #1

TIME:_____

ACTIVITY:_____

DURATION:_____ LEVEL_____

DISTANCE:_____

CALORIES BURNED:_____

ACTIVITY PULSE RATE:_____bpm

RECOVERY PULSE RATE:_____bpm

DIFFERENCE:_____

DAILY SLEEP TRACKER

TIME TO BED:_____

TIME UP:_____

HOURS OF SLEEP:_____

COMMENTS:_____

DAILY AB TRACKER

EXERCISE	SET X REPS X WGT
1._____	___X___X___
2._____	___X___X___
3._____	___X___X___
4._____	___X___X___
5._____	___X___X___

FITNESS CLASS
(or any physical activity-walk, jog, squash)

START:_____ FINISH:_____

TYPE:_____

INSTRUCTOR:_____

ESTIMATE OF
CALORIES BURNED:

COMMENTS:_____

CARDIO SESSION #2

TIME:_____

ACTIVITY:_____

DURATION:_____ LEVEL_____

DISTANCE:_____

CALORIES BURNED:_____

ACTIVITY PULSE RATE:_____bpm

RECOVERY PULSE RATE:_____bpm

DIFFERENCE:_____

COMMENTS:_____

TOTAL CALORIES
BURNED TODAY:

Daily Nutrition Tracking

NUTRITION	Points Goal	CAL option	PROT grams	FAT grams	CARB grams
Meal #1 – Time: H₂O____Cups(L)					
Meal #2 – Time: H₂O____Cups(L)					
Meal #3 – Time: H₂O____Cups(L)					
Meal #4 – Time: H₂O____Cups(L)					
Meal #5 – Time: H₂O____Cups(L)					
Meal #6 – Time: H₂O____Cups(L)					

1

Food Point Total For Today:		
Difference (Goal Points Minus Actual Points)		

Daily Totals: *(Add up each nutrient column. Convert each to calories. Add all and enter in "Total Calories")* — g   g   g

Conversion To Calories
*Multiply Total Grams of **Pro X 4** = Calories*
*Multiply Total Grams of **Carb X 4** = Calories*
*Multiply Total Grams of **Fat X 9** = Calories*

Total Calories — cal   cal   cal

Daily Percentages: *(Divide total calories of each nutrient by the Total Number of Calories)* — %   %   %

Total Calories Consumed:_____
                VS   **Difference**
Total Calories Burned: _____

Personal Training Log

	WEIGHT TRAINING	CARDIO SESSION #1

WEIGHT TRAINING

Date:_____ Phase:_____
Start:_____ Finish:_____ Duration:_____
Day:_____ Warm Up:_____

EXERCISE	SET X REPS X WEIGHT @ TEMPO
1.	___X___X_____ @__/__/__
	___X___X_____ @__/__/__
	___X___X_____ @__/__/__
	___X___X_____ @__/__/__
	___X___X_____ @__/__/__
2.	___X___X_____ @__/__/__
	___X___X_____ @__/__/__
	___X___X_____ @__/__/__
	___X___X_____ @__/__/__
	___X___X_____ @__/__/__
3.	___X___X_____ @__/__/__
	___X___X_____ @__/__/__
	___X___X_____ @__/__/__
	___X___X_____ @__/__/__
	___X___X_____ @__/__/__
4.	___X___X_____ @__/__/__
	___X___X_____ @__/__/__
	___X___X_____ @__/__/__
	___X___X_____ @__/__/__
	___X___X_____ @__/__/__
5.	___X___X_____ @__/__/__
	___X___X_____ @__/__/__
	___X___X_____ @__/__/__
	___X___X_____ @__/__/__
	___X___X_____ @__/__/__
6.	___X___X_____ @__/__/__
	___X___X_____ @__/__/__
	___X___X_____ @__/__/__
	___X___X_____ @__/__/__
	___X___X_____ @__/__/__
7.	___X___X_____ @__/__/__
	___X___X_____ @__/__/__
	___X___X_____ @__/__/__
	___X___X_____ @__/__/__
	___X___X_____ @__/__/__
8.	___X___X_____ @__/__/__
	___X___X_____ @__/__/__
	___X___X_____ @__/__/__
	___X___X_____ @__/__/__
	___X___X_____ @__/__/__
9.	___X___X_____ @__/__/__
	___X___X_____ @__/__/__
	___X___X_____ @__/__/__
	___X___X_____ @__/__/__
	___X___X_____ @__/__/__

CARDIO SESSION #1

TIME:_____
ACTIVITY:_____
DURATION:_____ LEVEL_____
DISTANCE:_____
CALORIES BURNED:_____
ACTIVITY PULSE RATE:_____bpm
RECOVERY PULSE RATE:_____bpm
DIFFERENCE:

DAILY SLEEP TRACKER

TIME TO BED:_____
TIME UP:_____
HOURS OF SLEEP:_____
COMMENTS:_____

DAILY AB TRACKER

EXERCISE	SET X REPS X WGT
1._____	___X___X____
2._____	___X___X____
3._____	___X___X____
4._____	___X___X____
5._____	___X___X____

FITNESS CLASS
(or any physical activity-walk, jog, squash)

START:_____ FINISH:_____
TYPE:_____
INSTRUCTOR:_____
ESTIMATE OF
CALORIES BURNED: [ ]
COMMENTS:_____

CARDIO SESSION #2

TIME:_____
ACTIVITY:_____
DURATION:_____ LEVEL_____
DISTANCE:_____
CALORIES BURNED:_____
ACTIVITY PULSE RATE:_____bpm
RECOVERY PULSE RATE:_____bpm
DIFFERENCE:_____

COMMENTS:_____

TOTAL CALORIES
BURNED TODAY: [ ]

1

NUTRITION	Points Goal	CAL *option*	PROT *grams*	FAT *grams*	CARB *grams*
Meal #1 – Time: H_2O_____Cups(L)					
Meal #2 – Time: H_2O_____Cups(L)					
Meal #3 – Time: H_2O_____Cups(L)					
Meal #4 – Time: H_2O_____Cups(L)					
Meal #5 – Time: H_2O_____Cups(L)					
Meal #6 – Time: H_2O_____Cups(L)					

1

Food Point Total For Today:					
Difference (Goal Points Minus Actual Points)					
Daily Totals: (*Add up each nutrient column. Convert each to calories. Add all and enter in "Total Calories"*)			*g*	*g*	*g*
Conversion To Calories Multiply Total Grams of **Pro X 4** = Calories Multiply Total Grams of **Carb X 4**=Calories Multiply Total Grams of **Fat X 9** = Calories	**Total Calories**		*cal*	*cal*	*cal*
Daily Percentages: (*Divide total calories of each nutrient by the Total Number of Calories*)			___ *%*	___ *%*	___ *%*

Total Calories Consumed:_____

VS   *Difference*

Total Calories Burned: _____

Personal Training Log

WEIGHT TRAINING

Date:_____Phase:_____

Start:_____Finish:_____Duration:_____

Day:_____Warm Up:_____

EXERCISE	SET X REPS X WEIGHT @ TEMPO
1.	___X___X _____ @__/__/__
	___X___X _____ @__/__/__
	___X___X _____ @__/__/__
	___X___X _____ @__/__/__
	___X___X _____ @__/__/__
2.	___X___X _____ @__/__/__
	___X___X _____ @__/__/__
	___X___X _____ @__/__/__
	___X___X _____ @__/__/__
	___X___X _____ @__/__/__
3.	___X___X _____ @__/__/__
	___X___X _____ @__/__/__
	___X___X _____ @__/__/__
	___X___X _____ @__/__/__
	___X___X _____ @__/__/__
4.	___X___X _____ @__/__/__
	___X___X _____ @__/__/__
	___X___X _____ @__/__/__
	___X___X _____ @__/__/__
	___X___X _____ @__/__/__
5.	___X___X _____ @__/__/__
	___X___X _____ @__/__/__
	___X___X _____ @__/__/__
	___X___X _____ @__/__/__
	___X___X _____ @__/__/__
6.	___X___X _____ @__/__/__
	___X___X _____ @__/__/__
	___X___X _____ @__/__/__
	___X___X _____ @__/__/__
	___X___X _____ @__/__/__
7.	___X___X _____ @__/__/__
	___X___X _____ @__/__/__
	___X___X _____ @__/__/__
	___X___X _____ @__/__/__
	___X___X _____ @__/__/__
8.	___X___X _____ @__/__/__
	___X___X _____ @__/__/__
	___X___X _____ @__/__/__
	___X___X _____ @__/__/__
	___X___X _____ @__/__/__
9.	___X___X _____ @__/__/__
	___X___X _____ @__/__/__
	___X___X _____ @__/__/__
	___X___X _____ @__/__/__
	___X___X _____ @__/__/__

CARDIO SESSION #1

TIME:_____

ACTIVITY:_____

DURATION:_____LEVEL_____

DISTANCE:_____

CALORIES BURNED:_____

ACTIVITY PULSE RATE:_____bpm

RECOVERY PULSE RATE:_____bpm

DIFFERENCE:

DAILY SLEEP TRACKER

TIME TO BED:_____

TIME UP:_____

HOURS OF SLEEP:_____

COMMENTS:_____

DAILY AB TRACKER

EXERCISE	SET X REPS X WGT
1._____	___X____X____
2._____	___X____X____
3._____	___X____X____
4._____	___X____X____
5._____	___X____X____

FITNESS CLASS
(or any physical activity-walk, jog, squash)

START:_____FINISH:_____

TYPE:_____

INSTRUCTOR:_____

ESTIMATE OF
CALORIES BURNED:

COMMENTS:_____

CARDIO SESSION #2

TIME:_____

ACTIVITY:_____

DURATION:_____LEVEL_____

DISTANCE:_____

CALORIES BURNED:_____

ACTIVITY PULSE RATE:_____bpm

RECOVERY PULSE RATE:_____bpm

DIFFERENCE: _____

COMMENTS:_____

TOTAL CALORIES
BURNED TODAY:

Daily Nutrition Tracking

NUTRITION	Points Goal	CAL *option*	PROT *grams*	FAT *grams*	CARB *grams*
Meal #1 – Time: H₂O____Cups(L)					
Meal #2 – Time: H₂O____Cups(L)					
Meal #3 – Time: H₂O____Cups(L)					
Meal #4 – Time: H₂O____Cups(L)					
Meal #5 – Time: H₂O____Cups(L)					
Meal #6 – Time: H₂O____Cups(L)					

1

Food Point Total For Today:				
Difference (Goal Points Minus Actual Points)				
Daily Totals: (Add up each nutrient column. Convert each to calories. Add all and enter in "Total Calories")		g	g	g
Conversion To Calories Multiply Total Grams of **Pro X 4** = Calories / Multiply Total Grams of **Carb X 4**=Calories / Multiply Total Grams of **Fat X 9** = Calories	**Total Calories**	cal	cal	cal
Daily Percentages: (Divide total calories of each nutrient by the Total Number of Calories)		%	%	%

Total Calories Consumed: _____
VS   *Difference*
Total Calories Burned: _____

Personal Training Log

<table>
<tr><td colspan="6">

WEIGHT TRAINING

Date:_____ Phase:_____

Start:_____ Finish:_____ Duration:_____

Day:_____ Warm Up:_____

</td></tr>
</table>

EXERCISE	SET X	REPS X	WEIGHT	@	TEMPO
1.	___X	___X	_____	@	_/_/_
	___X	___X	_____	@	_/_/_
	___X	___X	_____	@	_/_/_
	___X	___X	_____	@	_/_/_
	___X	___X	_____	@	_/_/_
2.	___X	___X	_____	@	_/_/_
	___X	___X	_____	@	_/_/_
	___X	___X	_____	@	_/_/_
	___X	___X	_____	@	_/_/_
	___X	___X	_____	@	_/_/_
3.	___X	___X	_____	@	_/_/_
	___X	___X	_____	@	_/_/_
	___X	___X	_____	@	_/_/_
	___X	___X	_____	@	_/_/_
	___X	___X	_____	@	_/_/_
4.	___X	___X	_____	@	_/_/_
	___X	___X	_____	@	_/_/_
	___X	___X	_____	@	_/_/_
	___X	___X	_____	@	_/_/_
	___X	___X	_____	@	_/_/_
5.	___X	___X	_____	@	_/_/_
	___X	___X	_____	@	_/_/_
	___X	___X	_____	@	_/_/_
	___X	___X	_____	@	_/_/_
	___X	___X	_____	@	_/_/_
6.	___X	___X	_____	@	_/_/_
	___X	___X	_____	@	_/_/_
	___X	___X	_____	@	_/_/_
	___X	___X	_____	@	_/_/_
	___X	___X	_____	@	_/_/_
7.	___X	___X	_____	@	_/_/_
	___X	___X	_____	@	_/_/_
	___X	___X	_____	@	_/_/_
	___X	___X	_____	@	_/_/_
	___X	___X	_____	@	_/_/_
8.	___X	___X	_____	@	_/_/_
	___X	___X	_____	@	_/_/_
	___X	___X	_____	@	_/_/_
	___X	___X	_____	@	_/_/_
	___X	___X	_____	@	_/_/_
9.	___X	___X	_____	@	_/_/_
	___X	___X	_____	@	_/_/_
	___X	___X	_____	@	_/_/_
	___X	___X	_____	@	_/_/_
	___X	___X	_____	@	_/_/_

CARDIO SESSION #1

TIME:_____

ACTIVITY:_____

DURATION:_____ LEVEL_____

DISTANCE:_____

CALORIES BURNED:_____

ACTIVITY PULSE RATE:_____ bpm

RECOVERY PULSE RATE:_____ bpm

DIFFERENCE:

DAILY SLEEP TRACKER

TIME TO BED:_____

TIME UP:_____

HOURS OF SLEEP:_____

COMMENTS:_____

DAILY AB TRACKER

EXERCISE	SET X	REPS X	WGT
1._____	___X	___X	_____
2._____	___X	___X	_____
3._____	___X	___X	_____
4._____	___X	___X	_____
5._____	___X	___X	_____

FITNESS CLASS
(or any physical activity-walk, jog, squash)

START:_____ FINISH:_____

TYPE:_____

INSTRUCTOR:_____

ESTIMATE OF
CALORIES BURNED: [____]

COMMENTS:_____

CARDIO SESSION #2

TIME:_____

ACTIVITY:_____

DURATION:_____ LEVEL_____

DISTANCE:_____

CALORIES BURNED:_____

ACTIVITY PULSE RATE:_____ bpm

RECOVERY PULSE RATE:_____ bpm

DIFFERENCE:_____

COMMENTS:_____

_____

TOTAL CALORIES
BURNED TODAY: [____]

1

Daily Nutrition Tracking

NUTRITION	Points Goal	CAL *option*	PROT *grams*	FAT *grams*	CARB *grams*
Meal #1 – Time: H$_2$O____Cups(L)					
Meal #2 – Time: H$_2$O____Cups(L)					
Meal #3 – Time: H$_2$O____Cups(L)					
Meal #4 – Time: H$_2$O____Cups(L)					
Meal #5 – Time: H$_2$O____Cups(L)					
Meal #6 – Time: H$_2$O____Cups(L)					

Food Point Total For Today:

Difference (Goal Points Minus Actual Points)

Daily Totals: (Add up each nutrient column. Convert each to calories. Add all and enter in "Total Calories") — g   g   g

Conversion To Calories
Multiply Total Grams of **Pro X 4** = Calories
Multiply Total Grams of **Carb X 4** = Calories
Multiply Total Grams of **Fat X 9** = Calories

Total Calories — cal   cal   cal

Daily Percentages: (Divide total calories of each nutrient by the Total Number of Calories) — %   %   %

Total Calories Consumed: _____
VS
Total Calories Burned: _____
Difference

Personal Training Log

WEIGHT TRAINING

Date:_____ Phase:_____

Start:_____ Finish:_____ Duration:_____

Day:_____ Warm Up:_____

EXERCISE	SET X REPS X WEIGHT @ TEMPO
1.	___X___X_____@__/__/__
	___X___X_____@__/__/__
	___X___X_____@__/__/__
	___X___X_____@__/__/__
	___X___X_____@__/__/__
2.	___X___X_____@__/__/__
	___X___X_____@__/__/__
	___X___X_____@__/__/__
	___X___X_____@__/__/__
	___X___X_____@__/__/__
3.	___X___X_____@__/__/__
	___X___X_____@__/__/__
	___X___X_____@__/__/__
	___X___X_____@__/__/__
	___X___X_____@__/__/__
4.	___X___X_____@__/__/__
	___X___X_____@__/__/__
	___X___X_____@__/__/__
	___X___X_____@__/__/__
	___X___X_____@__/__/__
5.	___X___X_____@__/__/__
	___X___X_____@__/__/__
	___X___X_____@__/__/__
	___X___X_____@__/__/__
	___X___X_____@__/__/__
6.	___X___X_____@__/__/__
	___X___X_____@__/__/__
	___X___X_____@__/__/__
	___X___X_____@__/__/__
	___X___X_____@__/__/__
7.	___X___X_____@__/__/__
	___X___X_____@__/__/__
	___X___X_____@__/__/__
	___X___X_____@__/__/__
	___X___X_____@__/__/__
8.	___X___X_____@__/__/__
	___X___X_____@__/__/__
	___X___X_____@__/__/__
	___X___X_____@__/__/__
	___X___X_____@__/__/__
9.	___X___X_____@__/__/__
	___X___X_____@__/__/__
	___X___X_____@__/__/__
	___X___X_____@__/__/__
	___X___X_____@__/__/__

CARDIO SESSION #1

TIME:_____

ACTIVITY:_____

DURATION:_____ LEVEL_____

DISTANCE:_____

CALORIES BURNED:_____

ACTIVITY PULSE RATE:_____bpm

RECOVERY PULSE RATE:_____bpm

DIFFERENCE:

DAILY SLEEP TRACKER

TIME TO BED:_____

TIME UP:_____

HOURS OF SLEEP:_____

COMMENTS:_____

DAILY AB TRACKER

	EXERCISE	SET X REPS X WGT
1._____		___X____X____
2._____		___X____X____
3._____		___X____X____
4._____		___X____X____
5._____		___X____X____

FITNESS CLASS

(or any physical activity-walk, jog, squash)

START:_____ FINISH:_____

TYPE:_____

INSTRUCTOR:_____

ESTIMATE OF
CALORIES BURNED:

COMMENTS:_____

CARDIO SESSION #2

TIME:_____

ACTIVITY:_____

DURATION:_____ LEVEL_____

DISTANCE:_____

CALORIES BURNED:_____

ACTIVITY PULSE RATE:_____bpm

RECOVERY PULSE RATE:_____bpm

DIFFERENCE:_____

COMMENTS:_____

_____

TOTAL CALORIES
BURNED TODAY:

Daily Nutrition Tracking

NUTRITION	Points Goal	CAL option	PROT grams	FAT grams	CARB grams
Meal #1 – Time: H₂O_____Cups(L)					
Meal #2 – Time: H₂O_____Cups(L)					
Meal #3 – Time: H₂O_____Cups(L)					
Meal #4 – Time: H₂O_____Cups(L)					
Meal #5 – Time: H₂O_____Cups(L)					
Meal #6 – Time: H₂O_____Cups(L)					

1

Food Point Total For Today:

Difference (Goal Points Minus Actual Points)

Daily Totals: (Add up each nutrient column. Convert each to calories. Add all and enter in "Total Calories")   **g   g   g**

Conversion To Calories
Multiply Total Grams of **Pro X 4** = Calories
Multiply Total Grams of **Carb X 4**=Calories
Multiply Total Grams of **Fat X 9** = Calories

Total Calories   **cal   cal   cal**

Daily Percentages: (Divide total calories of each nutrient by the Total Number of Calories)   **%   %   %**

***Total Calories Consumed:*_____**
           VS   ***Difference***
***Total Calories Burned:*_____**

WEIGHT TRAINING

Date:_____ Phase:_____

Start:_____ Finish:_____ Duration:_____

Day:_____ Warm Up:_____

EXERCISE	SET X REPS X WEIGHT @ TEMPO
1.	___X___X_____@__/__/__
	___X___X_____@__/__/__
	___X___X_____@__/__/__
	___X___X_____@__/__/__
	___X___X_____@__/__/__
2.	___X___X_____@__/__/__
	___X___X_____@__/__/__
	___X___X_____@__/__/__
	___X___X_____@__/__/__
	___X___X_____@__/__/__
3.	___X___X_____@__/__/__
	___X___X_____@__/__/__
	___X___X_____@__/__/__
	___X___X_____@__/__/__
	___X___X_____@__/__/__
4.	___X___X_____@__/__/__
	___X___X_____@__/__/__
	___X___X_____@__/__/__
	___X___X_____@__/__/__
	___X___X_____@__/__/__
5.	___X___X_____@__/__/__
	___X___X_____@__/__/__
	___X___X_____@__/__/__
	___X___X_____@__/__/__
	___X___X_____@__/__/__
6.	___X___X_____@__/__/__
	___X___X_____@__/__/__
	___X___X_____@__/__/__
	___X___X_____@__/__/__
	___X___X_____@__/__/__
7.	___X___X_____@__/__/__
	___X___X_____@__/__/__
	___X___X_____@__/__/__
	___X___X_____@__/__/__
	___X___X_____@__/__/__
8.	___X___X_____@__/__/__
	___X___X_____@__/__/__
	___X___X_____@__/__/__
	___X___X_____@__/__/__
	___X___X_____@__/__/__
9.	___X___X_____@__/__/__
	___X___X_____@__/__/__
	___X___X_____@__/__/__
	___X___X_____@__/__/__
	___X___X_____@__/__/__

CARDIO SESSION #1

TIME:_____

ACTIVITY:_____

DURATION:_____ LEVEL_____

DISTANCE:_____

CALORIES BURNED:_____

ACTIVITY PULSE RATE:_____ bpm

RECOVERY PULSE RATE:_____ bpm

DIFFERENCE:

DAILY SLEEP TRACKER

TIME TO BED:_____

TIME UP:_____

HOURS OF SLEEP:_____

COMMENTS:_____

DAILY AB TRACKER

EXERCISE	SET X REPS X WGT
1._____	___X___X____
2._____	___X___X____
3._____	___X___X____
4._____	___X___X____
5._____	___X___X____

FITNESS CLASS
(or any physical activity-walk, jog, squash)

START:_____ FINISH:_____

TYPE:_____

INSTRUCTOR:_____

ESTIMATE OF
CALORIES BURNED:

COMMENTS:_____

CARDIO SESSION #2

TIME:_____

ACTIVITY:_____

DURATION:_____ LEVEL_____

DISTANCE:_____

CALORIES BURNED:_____

ACTIVITY PULSE RATE:_____ bpm

RECOVERY PULSE RATE:_____ bpm

DIFFERENCE:_____

COMMENTS:_____

TOTAL CALORIES
BURNED TODAY:

NUTRITION	Points Goal	CAL *option*	PROT *grams*	FAT *grams*	CARB *grams*
Meal #1 – Time: H₂O____Cups(L)					
Meal #2 – Time: H₂O____Cups(L)					
Meal #3 – Time: H₂O____Cups(L)					
Meal #4 – Time: H₂O____Cups(L)					
Meal #5 – Time: H₂O____Cups(L)					
Meal #6 – Time: H₂O____Cups(L)					

Food Point Total For Today:

Difference (Goal Points Minus Actual Points)

Daily Totals: *(Add up each nutrient column. Convert each to calories. Add all and enter in "Total Calories")* — g   g   g

Conversion To Calories
Multiply Total Grams of **Pro X 4** = Calories
Multiply Total Grams of **Carb X 4**=Calories
Multiply Total Grams of **Fat X 9** = Calories

Total Calories — cal   cal   cal

Daily Percentages: (Divide total calories of each nutrient by the Total Number of Calories) — %   %   %

Total Calories Consumed:_____
                    VS   **Difference**
Total Calories Burned: _____

Personal Training Log

WEIGHT TRAINING

Date:_____ Phase:_____

Start:_____ Finish:_____ Duration:_____

Day:_____ Warm Up:_____

EXERCISE	SET X REPS X WEIGHT @ TEMPO
1.	___ X ___ X _____ @ __/__/__
	___ X ___ X _____ @ __/__/__
	___ X ___ X _____ @ __/__/__
	___ X ___ X _____ @ __/__/__
	___ X ___ X _____ @ __/__/__
2.	___ X ___ X _____ @ __/__/__
	___ X ___ X _____ @ __/__/__
	___ X ___ X _____ @ __/__/__
	___ X ___ X _____ @ __/__/__
	___ X ___ X _____ @ __/__/__
3.	___ X ___ X _____ @ __/__/__
	___ X ___ X _____ @ __/__/__
	___ X ___ X _____ @ __/__/__
	___ X ___ X _____ @ __/__/__
	___ X ___ X _____ @ __/__/__
4.	___ X ___ X _____ @ __/__/__
	___ X ___ X _____ @ __/__/__
	___ X ___ X _____ @ __/__/__
	___ X ___ X _____ @ __/__/__
	___ X ___ X _____ @ __/__/__
5.	___ X ___ X _____ @ __/__/__
	___ X ___ X _____ @ __/__/__
	___ X ___ X _____ @ __/__/__
	___ X ___ X _____ @ __/__/__
	___ X ___ X _____ @ __/__/__
6.	___ X ___ X _____ @ __/__/__
	___ X ___ X _____ @ __/__/__
	___ X ___ X _____ @ __/__/__
	___ X ___ X _____ @ __/__/__
	___ X ___ X _____ @ __/__/__
7.	___ X ___ X _____ @ __/__/__
	___ X ___ X _____ @ __/__/__
	___ X ___ X _____ @ __/__/__
	___ X ___ X _____ @ __/__/__
	___ X ___ X _____ @ __/__/__
8.	___ X ___ X _____ @ __/__/__
	___ X ___ X _____ @ __/__/__
	___ X ___ X _____ @ __/__/__
	___ X ___ X _____ @ __/__/__
	___ X ___ X _____ @ __/__/__
9.	___ X ___ X _____ @ __/__/__
	___ X ___ X _____ @ __/__/__
	___ X ___ X _____ @ __/__/__
	___ X ___ X _____ @ __/__/__
	___ X ___ X _____ @ __/__/__

CARDIO SESSION #1

TIME:_____

ACTIVITY:_____

DURATION:_____ LEVEL_____

DISTANCE:_____

CALORIES BURNED:_____

ACTIVITY PULSE RATE:_____ bpm

RECOVERY PULSE RATE:_____ bpm

DIFFERENCE:

DAILY SLEEP TRACKER

TIME TO BED:_____

TIME UP:_____

HOURS OF SLEEP:_____

COMMENTS:_____

DAILY AB TRACKER

EXERCISE	SET X REPS X WGT
1._____	___ X ___ X _____
2._____	___ X ___ X _____
3._____	___ X ___ X _____
4._____	___ X ___ X _____
5._____	___ X ___ X _____

FITNESS CLASS
(or any physical activity-walk, jog, squash)

START:_____ FINISH:_____

TYPE:_____

INSTRUCTOR:_____

ESTIMATE OF
CALORIES BURNED:

COMMENTS:_____

CARDIO SESSION #2

TIME:_____

ACTIVITY:_____

DURATION:_____ LEVEL_____

DISTANCE:_____

CALORIES BURNED:_____

ACTIVITY PULSE RATE:_____ bpm

RECOVERY PULSE RATE:_____ bpm

DIFFERENCE:_____

COMMENTS:_____

_____

TOTAL CALORIES
BURNED TODAY:

NUTRITION	Points Goal	CAL *option*	PROT *grams*	FAT *grams*	CARB *grams*
Meal #1 – Time: H₂O_____Cups(L)					
Meal #2 – Time: H₂O_____Cups(L)					
Meal #3 – Time: H₂O_____Cups(L)					
Meal #4 – Time: H₂O_____Cups(L)					
Meal #5 – Time: H₂O_____Cups(L)					
Meal #6 – Time: H₂O_____Cups(L)					
Food Point Total For Today:					
Difference *(Goal Points Minus Actual Points)*					
Daily Totals: *(Add up each nutrient column. Convert each to calories. Add all and enter in "Total Calories")*			*g*	*g*	*g*
Conversion To Calories Multiply Total Grams of **Pro X 4** = Calories / Multiply Total Grams of **Carb X 4** = Calories / Multiply Total Grams of **Fat X 9** = Calories	**Total Calories**		*cal*	*cal*	*cal*
Daily Percentages: *(Divide total calories of each nutrient by the Total Number of Calories)*			___ *%*	___ *%*	___ *%*

Total Calories Consumed:_____

VS   **Difference**

Total Calories Burned: _____

1

Personal Training Log

WEIGHT TRAINING

Date:_____ Phase:_____

Start:_____ Finish:_____ Duration:_____

Day:_____ Warm Up:_____

EXERCISE	SET X REPS X WEIGHT @ TEMPO
1.	___ X ___ X _____ @___/___/___
	___ X ___ X _____ @___/___/___
	___ X ___ X _____ @___/___/___
	___ X ___ X _____ @___/___/___
	___ X ___ X _____ @___/___/___
2.	___ X ___ X _____ @___/___/___
	___ X ___ X _____ @___/___/___
	___ X ___ X _____ @___/___/___
	___ X ___ X _____ @___/___/___
	___ X ___ X _____ @___/___/___
3.	___ X ___ X _____ @___/___/___
	___ X ___ X _____ @___/___/___
	___ X ___ X _____ @___/___/___
	___ X ___ X _____ @___/___/___
	___ X ___ X _____ @___/___/___
4.	___ X ___ X _____ @___/___/___
	___ X ___ X _____ @___/___/___
	___ X ___ X _____ @___/___/___
	___ X ___ X _____ @___/___/___
	___ X ___ X _____ @___/___/___
5.	___ X ___ X _____ @___/___/___
	___ X ___ X _____ @___/___/___
	___ X ___ X _____ @___/___/___
	___ X ___ X _____ @___/___/___
	___ X ___ X _____ @___/___/___
6.	___ X ___ X _____ @___/___/___
	___ X ___ X _____ @___/___/___
	___ X ___ X _____ @___/___/___
	___ X ___ X _____ @___/___/___
	___ X ___ X _____ @___/___/___
7.	___ X ___ X _____ @___/___/___
	___ X ___ X _____ @___/___/___
	___ X ___ X _____ @___/___/___
	___ X ___ X _____ @___/___/___
	___ X ___ X _____ @___/___/___
8.	___ X ___ X _____ @___/___/___
	___ X ___ X _____ @___/___/___
	___ X ___ X _____ @___/___/___
	___ X ___ X _____ @___/___/___
	___ X ___ X _____ @___/___/___
9.	___ X ___ X _____ @___/___/___
	___ X ___ X _____ @___/___/___
	___ X ___ X _____ @___/___/___
	___ X ___ X _____ @___/___/___
	___ X ___ X _____ @___/___/___

CARDIO SESSION #1

TIME:_____

ACTIVITY:_____

DURATION:_____ LEVEL_____

DISTANCE:_____

CALORIES BURNED:_____

ACTIVITY PULSE RATE:_____bpm

RECOVERY PULSE RATE:_____bpm

DIFFERENCE:

DAILY SLEEP TRACKER

TIME TO BED:_____

TIME UP:_____

HOURS OF SLEEP:_____

COMMENTS:_____

DAILY AB TRACKER

EXERCISE	SET X REPS X WGT
1._____	___ X ___ X ___
2._____	___ X ___ X ___
3._____	___ X ___ X ___
4._____	___ X ___ X ___
5._____	___ X ___ X ___

FITNESS CLASS
(or any physical activity-walk, jog, squash)

START:_____ FINISH:_____

TYPE:_____

INSTRUCTOR:_____

ESTIMATE OF
CALORIES BURNED: [____]

COMMENTS:_____

CARDIO SESSION #2

TIME:_____

ACTIVITY:_____

DURATION:_____ LEVEL_____

DISTANCE:_____

CALORIES BURNED:_____

ACTIVITY PULSE RATE:_____bpm

RECOVERY PULSE RATE:_____bpm

DIFFERENCE:_____

COMMENTS:_____

TOTAL CALORIES
BURNED TODAY: [____]

1

Daily Nutrition Tracking

NUTRITION	Points Goal	CAL *option*	PROT *grams*	FAT *grams*	CARB *grams*
Meal #1 – Time: H₂O____Cups(L)					
Meal #2 – Time: H₂O____Cups(L)					
Meal #3 – Time: H₂O____Cups(L)					
Meal #4 – Time: H₂O____Cups(L)					
Meal #5 – Time: H₂O____Cups(L)					
Meal #6 – Time: H₂O____Cups(L)					
Food Point Total For Today:					
Difference (Goal Points Minus Actual Points)					

Daily Totals: *(Add up each nutrient column. Convert each to calories. Add all and enter in "Total Calories")* — g g g

Conversion To Calories
Multiply Total Grams of **Pro X 4** = Calories
Multiply Total Grams of **Carb X 4** = Calories
Multiply Total Grams of **Fat X 9** = Calories

Total Calories — cal cal cal

Daily Percentages: *(Divide total calories of each nutrient by the Total Number of Calories)* — % % %

Total Calories Consumed:_____
VS   **Difference**
Total Calories Burned: _____

Personal Training Log

WEIGHT TRAINING

Date:_____ Phase:_____

Start:_____ Finish:_____ Duration:_____

Day:_____ Warm Up:_____

EXERCISE	SET X REPS X WEIGHT @ TEMPO
1.	___X___X_____ @__/__/__
	___X___X_____ @__/__/__
	___X___X_____ @__/__/__
	___X___X_____ @__/__/__
	___X___X_____ @__/__/__
2.	___X___X_____ @__/__/__
	___X___X_____ @__/__/__
	___X___X_____ @__/__/__
	___X___X_____ @__/__/__
	___X___X_____ @__/__/__
3.	___X___X_____ @__/__/__
	___X___X_____ @__/__/__
	___X___X_____ @__/__/__
	___X___X_____ @__/__/__
	___X___X_____ @__/__/__
4.	___X___X_____ @__/__/__
	___X___X_____ @__/__/__
	___X___X_____ @__/__/__
	___X___X_____ @__/__/__
	___X___X_____ @__/__/__
5.	___X___X_____ @__/__/__
	___X___X_____ @__/__/__
	___X___X_____ @__/__/__
	___X___X_____ @__/__/__
	___X___X_____ @__/__/__
6.	___X___X_____ @__/__/__
	___X___X_____ @__/__/__
	___X___X_____ @__/__/__
	___X___X_____ @__/__/__
	___X___X_____ @__/__/__
7.	___X___X_____ @__/__/__
	___X___X_____ @__/__/__
	___X___X_____ @__/__/__
	___X___X_____ @__/__/__
	___X___X_____ @__/__/__
8.	___X___X_____ @__/__/__
	___X___X_____ @__/__/__
	___X___X_____ @__/__/__
	___X___X_____ @__/__/__
	___X___X_____ @__/__/__
9.	___X___X_____ @__/__/__
	___X___X_____ @__/__/__
	___X___X_____ @__/__/__
	___X___X_____ @__/__/__
	___X___X_____ @__/__/__

1

CARDIO SESSION #1

TIME:_____

ACTIVITY:_____

DURATION:_____LEVEL_____

DISTANCE:_____

CALORIES BURNED:_____

ACTIVITY PULSE RATE:_____bpm

RECOVERY PULSE RATE:_____bpm

DIFFERENCE:

DAILY SLEEP TRACKER

TIME TO BED:_____

TIME UP:_____

HOURS OF SLEEP:_____

COMMENTS:_____

DAILY AB TRACKER

EXERCISE	SET X REPS X WGT
1._____	___X___X___
2._____	___X___X___
3._____	___X___X___
4._____	___X___X___
5._____	___X___X___

FITNESS CLASS
(or any physical activity-walk, jog, squash)

START:_____FINISH:_____

TYPE:_____

INSTRUCTOR:_____

ESTIMATE OF
CALORIES BURNED: [ ]

COMMENTS:_____

CARDIO SESSION #2

TIME:_____

ACTIVITY:_____

DURATION:_____LEVEL_____

DISTANCE:_____

CALORIES BURNED:_____

ACTIVITY PULSE RATE:_____bpm

RECOVERY PULSE RATE:_____bpm

DIFFERENCE:_____

COMMENTS:_____

_____

TOTAL CALORIES
BURNED TODAY: [ ]

Daily Nutrition Tracking

NUTRITION	Points Goal	CAL option	PROT grams	FAT grams	CARB grams
Meal #1 – Time: H₂O____Cups(L)					
Meal #2 – Time: H₂O____Cups(L)					
Meal #3 – Time: H₂O____Cups(L)					
Meal #4 – Time: H₂O____Cups(L)					
Meal #5 – Time: H₂O____Cups(L)					
Meal #6 – Time: H₂O____Cups(L)					

Food Point Total For Today:

Difference (Goal Points Minus Actual Points)

Daily Totals: (Add up each nutrient column. Convert each to calories. Add all and enter in "Total Calories") — g   g   g

Conversion To Calories
Multiply Total Grams of **Pro X 4** = Calories
Multiply Total Grams of **Carb X 4** = Calories
Multiply Total Grams of **Fat X 9** = Calories

Total Calories — cal   cal   cal

Daily Percentages: (Divide total calories of each nutrient by the Total Number of Calories) — %   %   %

Total Calories Consumed:_____
VS
Total Calories Burned: _____
Difference

1

Personal Training Log

WEIGHT TRAINING

Date:_____ Phase:_____

Start:_____ Finish:_____ Duration:_____

Day:_____ Warm Up:_____

EXERCISE	SET X REPS X WEIGHT @ TEMPO
1.	___X___X_____ @__/__/__
	___X___X_____ @__/__/__
	___X___X_____ @__/__/__
	___X___X_____ @__/__/__
	___X___X_____ @__/__/__
2.	___X___X_____ @__/__/__
	___X___X_____ @__/__/__
	___X___X_____ @__/__/__
	___X___X_____ @__/__/__
	___X___X_____ @__/__/__
3.	___X___X_____ @__/__/__
	___X___X_____ @__/__/__
	___X___X_____ @__/__/__
	___X___X_____ @__/__/__
	___X___X_____ @__/__/__
4.	___X___X_____ @__/__/__
	___X___X_____ @__/__/__
	___X___X_____ @__/__/__
	___X___X_____ @__/__/__
	___X___X_____ @__/__/__
5.	___X___X_____ @__/__/__
	___X___X_____ @__/__/__
	___X___X_____ @__/__/__
	___X___X_____ @__/__/__
	___X___X_____ @__/__/__
6.	___X___X_____ @__/__/__
	___X___X_____ @__/__/__
	___X___X_____ @__/__/__
	___X___X_____ @__/__/__
	___X___X_____ @__/__/__
7.	___X___X_____ @__/__/__
	___X___X_____ @__/__/__
	___X___X_____ @__/__/__
	___X___X_____ @__/__/__
	___X___X_____ @__/__/__
8.	___X___X_____ @__/__/__
	___X___X_____ @__/__/__
	___X___X_____ @__/__/__
	___X___X_____ @__/__/__
	___X___X_____ @__/__/__
9.	___X___X_____ @__/__/__
	___X___X_____ @__/__/__
	___X___X_____ @__/__/__
	___X___X_____ @__/__/__
	___X___X_____ @__/__/__

CARDIO SESSION #1

TIME:_____

ACTIVITY:_____

DURATION:_____ LEVEL_____

DISTANCE:_____

CALORIES BURNED:_____

ACTIVITY PULSE RATE:_____bpm

RECOVERY PULSE RATE:_____bpm

DIFFERENCE:

DAILY SLEEP TRACKER

TIME TO BED:_____

TIME UP:_____

HOURS OF SLEEP:_____

COMMENTS:_____

DAILY AB TRACKER

EXERCISE	SET X REPS X WGT
1._____	___X___X_____
2._____	___X___X_____
3._____	___X___X_____
4._____	___X___X_____
5._____	___X___X_____

FITNESS CLASS
(or any physical activity-walk, jog, squash)

START:_____ FINISH:_____

TYPE:_____

INSTRUCTOR:_____

ESTIMATE OF
CALORIES BURNED:

COMMENTS:_____

CARDIO SESSION #2

TIME:_____

ACTIVITY:_____

DURATION:_____ LEVEL_____

DISTANCE:_____

CALORIES BURNED:_____

ACTIVITY PULSE RATE:_____bpm

RECOVERY PULSE RATE:_____bpm

DIFFERENCE:_____

COMMENTS:_____

TOTAL CALORIES
BURNED TODAY:

Daily Nutrition Tracking

NUTRITION	Points Goal	CAL *option*	PROT *grams*	FAT *grams*	CARB *grams*
Meal #1 – Time:　　　　H₂O＿＿Cups(L)					
Meal #2 – Time:　　　　H₂O＿＿Cups(L)					
Meal #3 – Time:　　　　H₂O＿＿Cups(L)					
Meal #4 – Time:　　　　H₂O＿＿Cups(L)					
Meal #5 – Time:　　　　H₂O＿＿Cups(L)					
Meal #6 – Time:　　　　H₂O＿＿Cups(L)					
Food Point Total For Today:					
Difference (Goal Points Minus Actual Points)					
Daily Totals: (Add up each nutrient column. Convert each to calories. Add all and enter in "Total Calories")			g	g	g
Conversion To Calories Multiply Total Grams of **Pro X 4** = Calories / Multiply Total Grams of **Carb X 4** = Calories / Multiply Total Grams of **Fat X 9** = Calories — ***Total Calories***			cal	cal	cal
Daily Percentages: (Divide total calories of each nutrient by the Total Number of Calories)			＿%	＿%	＿%
Total Calories Consumed:＿＿＿ / ***VS*** / ***Total Calories Burned:***＿＿＿　　***Difference***					

1

Personal Training Log

WEIGHT TRAINING

Date:_____ Phase:_____
Start:_____ Finish:_____ Duration:_____
Day:_____ Warm Up:_____

EXERCISE	SET X REPS X WEIGHT @ TEMPO
1.	___ X ___ X _____ @ __/__/__
	___ X ___ X _____ @ __/__/__
	___ X ___ X _____ @ __/__/__
	___ X ___ X _____ @ __/__/__
	___ X ___ X _____ @ __/__/__
2.	___ X ___ X _____ @ __/__/__
	___ X ___ X _____ @ __/__/__
	___ X ___ X _____ @ __/__/__
	___ X ___ X _____ @ __/__/__
	___ X ___ X _____ @ __/__/__
3.	___ X ___ X _____ @ __/__/__
	___ X ___ X _____ @ __/__/__
	___ X ___ X _____ @ __/__/__
	___ X ___ X _____ @ __/__/__
	___ X ___ X _____ @ __/__/__
4.	___ X ___ X _____ @ __/__/__
	___ X ___ X _____ @ __/__/__
	___ X ___ X _____ @ __/__/__
	___ X ___ X _____ @ __/__/__
	___ X ___ X _____ @ __/__/__
5.	___ X ___ X _____ @ __/__/__
	___ X ___ X _____ @ __/__/__
	___ X ___ X _____ @ __/__/__
	___ X ___ X _____ @ __/__/__
	___ X ___ X _____ @ __/__/__
6.	___ X ___ X _____ @ __/__/__
	___ X ___ X _____ @ __/__/__
	___ X ___ X _____ @ __/__/__
	___ X ___ X _____ @ __/__/__
	___ X ___ X _____ @ __/__/__
7.	___ X ___ X _____ @ __/__/__
	___ X ___ X _____ @ __/__/__
	___ X ___ X _____ @ __/__/__
	___ X ___ X _____ @ __/__/__
	___ X ___ X _____ @ __/__/__
8.	___ X ___ X _____ @ __/__/__
	___ X ___ X _____ @ __/__/__
	___ X ___ X _____ @ __/__/__
	___ X ___ X _____ @ __/__/__
	___ X ___ X _____ @ __/__/__
9.	___ X ___ X _____ @ __/__/__
	___ X ___ X _____ @ __/__/__
	___ X ___ X _____ @ __/__/__
	___ X ___ X _____ @ __/__/__
	___ X ___ X _____ @ __/__/__

CARDIO SESSION #1

TIME:_____
ACTIVITY:_____
DURATION:_____ LEVEL_____
DISTANCE:_____
CALORIES BURNED:_____
ACTIVITY PULSE RATE:_____ bpm
RECOVERY PULSE RATE:_____ bpm
DIFFERENCE:

DAILY SLEEP TRACKER

TIME TO BED:_____
TIME UP:_____
HOURS OF SLEEP:_____
COMMENTS:_____

DAILY AB TRACKER

EXERCISE	SET X REPS X WGT
1._____	___ X ___ X _____
2._____	___ X ___ X _____
3._____	___ X ___ X _____
4._____	___ X ___ X _____
5._____	___ X ___ X _____

FITNESS CLASS

(or any physical activity-walk, jog, squash)

START:_____ FINISH:_____
TYPE:_____
INSTRUCTOR:_____
ESTIMATE OF
CALORIES BURNED:
COMMENTS:_____

CARDIO SESSION #2

TIME:_____
ACTIVITY:_____
DURATION:_____ LEVEL_____
DISTANCE:_____
CALORIES BURNED:_____
ACTIVITY PULSE RATE:_____ bpm
RECOVERY PULSE RATE:_____ bpm
DIFFERENCE:_____

COMMENTS:_____

TOTAL CALORIES
BURNED TODAY:

NUTRITION			Points Goal	CAL *option*	PROT *grams*	FAT *grams*	CARB *grams*
Meal #1 – Time:	H₂O___Cups(L)						
Meal #2 – Time:	H₂O___Cups(L)						
Meal #3 – Time:	H₂O___Cups(L)						
Meal #4 – Time:	H₂O___Cups(L)						
Meal #5 – Time:	H₂O___Cups(L)						
Meal #6 – Time:	H₂O___Cups(L)						

Food Point Total For Today:			
Difference (Goal Points Minus Actual Points)			

Daily Totals: *(Add up each nutrient column. Convert each to calories. Add all and enter in "Total Calories")* — g   g   g

Conversion To Calories
Multiply Total Grams of **Pro X 4** = Calories
Multiply Total Grams of **Carb X 4** = Calories
Multiply Total Grams of **Fat X 9** = Calories

Total Calories — cal   cal   cal

Daily Percentages: (Divide total calories of each nutrient by the Total Number of Calories) — %   %   %

Total Calories Consumed:_____
          VS   *Difference*
Total Calories Burned: _____

1

Progress Evaluation

Did you meet your goals for this cycle? Yes ☐ No ☐

If not, what prevented you from reaching your goals?

_____

_____

_____

_____

State the positive changes that occurred during this cycle even if you didn't meet all your goals:

_____

_____

_____

_____

What do you plan to do differently during the next cycle?

_____

_____

_____

Personal Trainers/Teachers Evaluation

_____

_____

_____

_____

_____

_____

_____

Enter Cycle

2

Personal Fitness Evaluation

Date:_____Height:_____Weight:_____Age:_____

Medical History:_____

_____

TESTING:

Resting Heart Rate:_____bpm   Blood Pressure:____/____   Body Fat:____%

Flexibility:_____   Push Ups:_____   Sit Ups:_____   Chin Ups:_____

Other Required Tests & Results:

1._____ [ ]   2._____ [ ]   3._____ [ ]

4._____ [ ]   5._____ [ ]   6._____ [ ]

WAIST TO HIP RATIO:

Waist:_____ Divided by Hips:_____ = [   ]   Women: 0.8 or less
                                                            Men: 0.95 or less

GOALS FOR THIS CYCLE:

1._____   3._____

2._____   4._____

YOUR PLAN TO ACHIEVE YOUR GOALS:

Be very specific in your plan, for example you may want to increase your cardio sessions from 20 to 25 minutes or you may want to increase your daily water intake by 1 glass. State this in your plan. Be careful to make your goals REALISTIC and ATTAINABLE. Keep in mind you do not have to use all five spaces provided. Keep it simple!

1._____

2._____

3._____

4._____

5._____

Weight Training Program:

	Day 1	Tempo		Day 2	Tempo
1.	_____	_/_/_	1.	_____	_/_/_
2.	_____	_/_/_	2.	_____	_/_/_
3.	_____	_/_/_	3.	_____	_/_/_
4.	_____	_/_/_	4.	_____	_/_/_
5.	_____	_/_/_	5.	_____	_/_/_
6.	_____	_/_/_	6.	_____	_/_/_
7.	_____	_/_/_	7.	_____	_/_/_
8.	_____	_/_/_	8.	_____	_/_/_
9.	_____	_/_/_	9.	_____	_/_/_

Aerobic Exercise Plan:

Type:_____ ___to___ x per week @____ to____min/session

Suggested Training Heart Rate: _____ to_____ beats/min

Aerobic Class Recommendation: _____

Current Eating Habits
(Typical Day)

Breakfast:_____
Snack:_____
Lunch: _____
Snack:_____
Dinner:_____
Evening Snack: _____

Suggested Changes to Eating Habits

Meal 1:_____

Meal 2: _____

Meal 3: _____

Meal 4: _____

Meal 5: _____

Meal 6: _____

Photograph - Start

Date Photograph taken: _____

Weight: _____ % Body Fat: _____

2

PLACE PHOTO
HERE

Photograph - End of Cycle #2

Date Photograph taken: _____

Weight: _____ % Body Fat: _____

PLACE PHOTO
HERE

2

Personal Training Log

WEIGHT TRAINING

Date:_____Phase:_____

Start:_____Finish:_____Duration:_____

Day:_____Warm Up:_____

EXERCISE	SET X REPS X WEIGHT @ TEMPO
1.	___X___X_____@__/__/__ ___X___X_____@__/__/__ ___X___X_____@__/__/__ ___X___X_____@__/__/__ ___X___X_____@__/__/__
2.	___X___X_____@__/__/__ ___X___X_____@__/__/__ ___X___X_____@__/__/__ ___X___X_____@__/__/__ ___X___X_____@__/__/__
3.	___X___X_____@__/__/__ ___X___X_____@__/__/__ ___X___X_____@__/__/__ ___X___X_____@__/__/__ ___X___X_____@__/__/__
4.	___X___X_____@__/__/__ ___X___X_____@__/__/__ ___X___X_____@__/__/__ ___X___X_____@__/__/__ ___X___X_____@__/__/__
5.	___X___X_____@__/__/__ ___X___X_____@__/__/__ ___X___X_____@__/__/__ ___X___X_____@__/__/__ ___X___X_____@__/__/__
6.	___X___X_____@__/__/__ ___X___X_____@__/__/__ ___X___X_____@__/__/__ ___X___X_____@__/__/__ ___X___X_____@__/__/__
7.	___X___X_____@__/__/__ ___X___X_____@__/__/__ ___X___X_____@__/__/__ ___X___X_____@__/__/__ ___X___X_____@__/__/__
8.	___X___X_____@__/__/__ ___X___X_____@__/__/__ ___X___X_____@__/__/__ ___X___X_____@__/__/__ ___X___X_____@__/__/__
9.	___X___X_____@__/__/__ ___X___X_____@__/__/__ ___X___X_____@__/__/__ ___X___X_____@__/__/__ ___X___X_____@__/__/__

CARDIO SESSION #1

TIME:_____

ACTIVITY:_____

DURATION:_____LEVEL_____

DISTANCE:_____

CALORIES BURNED:_____

ACTIVITY PULSE RATE:_____bpm

RECOVERY PULSE RATE:_____bpm

DIFFERENCE:

DAILY SLEEP TRACKER

TIME TO BED:_____

TIME UP:_____

HOURS OF SLEEP:_____

COMMENTS:_____

DAILY AB TRACKER

EXERCISE	SET X REPS X WGT
1._____	___X___X_____
2._____	___X___X_____
3._____	___X___X_____
4._____	___X___X_____
5._____	___X___X_____

FITNESS CLASS
(or any physical activity-walk, jog, squash)

START:_____FINISH:_____

TYPE:_____

INSTRUCTOR:_____

ESTIMATE OF
CALORIES BURNED:

COMMENTS:_____

CARDIO SESSION #2

TIME:_____

ACTIVITY:_____

DURATION:_____LEVEL_____

DISTANCE:_____

CALORIES BURNED:_____

ACTIVITY PULSE RATE:_____bpm

RECOVERY PULSE RATE:_____bpm

DIFFERENCE:_____

COMMENTS:_____

TOTAL CALORIES
BURNED TODAY:

2

NUTRITION	Points Goal	CAL *option*	PROT *grams*	FAT *grams*	CARB *grams*
Meal #1 – Time: H₂O_____Cups(L)					
Meal #2 – Time: H₂O_____Cups(L)					
Meal #3 – Time: H₂O_____Cups(L)					
Meal #4 – Time: H₂O_____Cups(L)					
Meal #5 – Time: H₂O_____Cups(L)					
Meal #6 – Time: H₂O_____Cups(L)					
Food Point Total For Today:					
Difference (Goal Points Minus Actual Points)					
Daily Totals: (Add up each nutrient column. Convert each to calories. Add all and enter in "Total Calories")			g	g	g
Conversion To Calories Multiply Total Grams of **Pro X 4** = Calories Multiply Total Grams of **Carb X 4** = Calories Multiply Total Grams of **Fat X 9** = Calories	**Total Calories**		cal	cal	cal
Daily Percentages: (Divide total calories of each nutrient by the Total Number of Calories)			%	%	%

Total Calories Consumed: _____

VS   **Difference**

Total Calories Burned: _____

2

Personal Training Log

WEIGHT TRAINING

Date:_____ Phase:_____

Start:_____ Finish:_____ Duration:_____

Day:_____ Warm Up:_____

EXERCISE	SET X REPS X WEIGHT @ TEMPO
1.	___X___X_____@___/___/___
	___X___X_____@___/___/___
	___X___X_____@___/___/___
	___X___X_____@___/___/___
	___X___X_____@___/___/___
2.	___X___X_____@___/___/___
	___X___X_____@___/___/___
	___X___X_____@___/___/___
	___X___X_____@___/___/___
	___X___X_____@___/___/___
3.	___X___X_____@___/___/___
	___X___X_____@___/___/___
	___X___X_____@___/___/___
	___X___X_____@___/___/___
	___X___X_____@___/___/___
4.	___X___X_____@___/___/___
	___X___X_____@___/___/___
	___X___X_____@___/___/___
	___X___X_____@___/___/___
	___X___X_____@___/___/___
5.	___X___X_____@___/___/___
	___X___X_____@___/___/___
	___X___X_____@___/___/___
	___X___X_____@___/___/___
	___X___X_____@___/___/___
6.	___X___X_____@___/___/___
	___X___X_____@___/___/___
	___X___X_____@___/___/___
	___X___X_____@___/___/___
	___X___X_____@___/___/___
7.	___X___X_____@___/___/___
	___X___X_____@___/___/___
	___X___X_____@___/___/___
	___X___X_____@___/___/___
	___X___X_____@___/___/___
8.	___X___X_____@___/___/___
	___X___X_____@___/___/___
	___X___X_____@___/___/___
	___X___X_____@___/___/___
	___X___X_____@___/___/___
9.	___X___X_____@___/___/___
	___X___X_____@___/___/___
	___X___X_____@___/___/___
	___X___X_____@___/___/___
	___X___X_____@___/___/___

CARDIO SESSION #1

TIME:_____

ACTIVITY:_____

DURATION:_____ LEVEL_____

DISTANCE:_____

CALORIES BURNED:_____

ACTIVITY PULSE RATE:_____ bpm

RECOVERY PULSE RATE:_____ bpm

DIFFERENCE:

DAILY SLEEP TRACKER

TIME TO BED:_____

TIME UP:_____

HOURS OF SLEEP:_____

COMMENTS:_____

DAILY AB TRACKER

EXERCISE	SET X REPS X WGT
1._____	___X_____X_____
2._____	___X_____X_____
3._____	___X_____X_____
4._____	___X_____X_____
5._____	___X_____X_____

FITNESS CLASS
(or any physical activity-walk, jog, squash)

START:_____ FINISH:_____

TYPE:_____

INSTRUCTOR:_____

ESTIMATE OF
CALORIES BURNED:

COMMENTS:_____

CARDIO SESSION #2

TIME:_____

ACTIVITY:_____

DURATION:_____ LEVEL

DISTANCE:_____

CALORIES BURNED:_____

ACTIVITY PULSE RATE:_____ bpm

RECOVERY PULSE RATE:_____ bpm

DIFFERENCE:_____

COMMENTS:_____

TOTAL CALORIES
BURNED TODAY:

NUTRITION	Points Goal	CAL _option_	PROT _grams_	FAT _grams_	CARB _grams_
Meal #1 – Time: H₂O_____Cups(L)					
Meal #2 – Time: H₂O_____Cups(L)					
Meal #3 – Time: II₂O_____Cups(L)					
Meal #4 – Time: H₂O_____Cups(L)					
Meal #5 – Time: H₂O_____Cups(L)					
Meal #6 – Time: H₂O____Cups(L)					
**Food Point Total For Today:**					
**Difference** (Goal Points Minus Actual Points)					
**Daily Totals:** (Add up each nutrient column. Convert each to calories. Add all and enter in "Total Calories")			g	g	g
**Conversion To Calories** _Multiply Total Grams of **Pro X 4** = Calories_ _Multiply Total Grams of **Carb X 4**=Calories_ _Multiply Total Grams of **Fat X 9** = Calories_	_**Total Calories**_		cal	cal	cal
**Daily Percentages:** (Divide total calories of each nutrient by the Total Number of Calories)			%	%	%

2

Total Calories Consumed:_____

              VS   *Difference*

Total Calories Burned: _____

Personal Training Log

WEIGHT TRAINING

Date:_____ Phase:_____

Start:_____ Finish:_____ Duration:_____

Day:_____ Warm Up:_____

EXERCISE	SET X REPS X WEIGHT @ TEMPO
1.	___X___X_____@___/___/___
	___X___X_____@___/___/___
	___X___X_____@___/___/___
	___X___X_____@___/___/___
	___X___X_____@___/___/___
2.	___X___X_____@___/___/___
	___X___X_____@___/___/___
	___X___X_____@___/___/___
	___X___X_____@___/___/___
	___X___X_____@___/___/___
3.	___X___X_____@___/___/___
	___X___X_____@___/___/___
	___X___X_____@___/___/___
	___X___X_____@___/___/___
	___X___X_____@___/___/___
4.	___X___X_____@___/___/___
	___X___X_____@___/___/___
	___X___X_____@___/___/___
	___X___X_____@___/___/___
	___X___X_____@___/___/___
5.	___X___X_____@___/___/___
	___X___X_____@___/___/___
	___X___X_____@___/___/___
	___X___X_____@___/___/___
	___X___X_____@___/___/___
6.	___X___X_____@___/___/___
	___X___X_____@___/___/___
	___X___X_____@___/___/___
	___X___X_____@___/___/___
	___X___X_____@___/___/___
7.	___X___X_____@___/___/___
	___X___X_____@___/___/___
	___X___X_____@___/___/___
	___X___X_____@___/___/___
	___X___X_____@___/___/___
8.	___X___X_____@___/___/___
	___X___X_____@___/___/___
	___X___X_____@___/___/___
	___X___X_____@___/___/___
	___X___X_____@___/___/___
9.	___X___X_____@___/___/___
	___X___X_____@___/___/___
	___X___X_____@___/___/___
	___X___X_____@___/___/___
	___X___X_____@___/___/___

CARDIO SESSION #1

TIME:_____

ACTIVITY:_____

DURATION:_____ LEVEL_____

DISTANCE:_____

CALORIES BURNED:_____

ACTIVITY PULSE RATE:_____bpm

RECOVERY PULSE RATE:_____bpm

DIFFERENCE:

DAILY SLEEP TRACKER

TIME TO BED:_____

TIME UP:_____

HOURS OF SLEEP:_____

COMMENTS:_____

DAILY AB TRACKER

EXERCISE	SET X REPS X WGT
1._____	___X___X___
2._____	___X___X___
3._____	___X___X___
4._____	___X___X___
5._____	___X___X___

FITNESS CLASS
(or any physical activity-walk, jog, squash)

START:_____ FINISH:_____

TYPE:_____

INSTRUCTOR:_____

ESTIMATE OF
CALORIES BURNED: [ ]

COMMENTS:_____

CARDIO SESSION #2

TIME:_____

ACTIVITY:_____

DURATION:_____ LEVEL_____

DISTANCE:_____

CALORIES BURNED:_____

ACTIVITY PULSE RATE:_____bpm

RECOVERY PULSE RATE:_____bpm

DIFFERENCE:_____

COMMENTS:_____

TOTAL CALORIES
BURNED TODAY: [ ]

NUTRITION	Points Goal	CAL *option*	PROT *grams*	FAT *grams*	CARB *grams*
Meal #1 – Time: H₂O____Cups(L)					
Meal #2 – Time: H₂O____Cups(L)					
Meal #3 – Time: H₂O____Cups(L)					
Meal #4 – Time: H₂O____Cups(L)					
Meal #5 – Time: H₂O____Cups(L)					
Meal #6 – Time: H₂O____Cups(L)					

2

Food Point Total For Today:

Difference (Goal Points Minus Actual Points)

Daily Totals: (Add up each nutrient column. Convert each to calories. Add all and enter in "Total Calories")   **g** **g** **g**

Conversion To Calories
Multiply Total Grams of **Pro X 4** = Calories
Multiply Total Grams of **Carb X 4**=Calories
Multiply Total Grams of **Fat X 9** = Calories

Total Calories   **cal** **cal** **cal**

Daily Percentages: (Divide total calories of each nutrient by the Total Number of Calories)   **%** **%** **%**

Total Calories Consumed:_____
              VS   **Difference**
Total Calories Burned: _____

Personal Training Log

WEIGHT TRAINING

Date:_____ Phase:_____

Start:_____ Finish:_____ Duration:_____

Day:_____ Warm Up:_____

EXERCISE	SET X REPS X WEIGHT @ TEMPO
1.	___X___X___ @__/__/__
	___X___X___ @__/__/__
	___X___X___ @__/__/__
	___X___X___ @__/__/__
	___X___X___ @__/__/__
2.	___X___X___ @__/__/__
	___X___X___ @__/__/__
	___X___X___ @__/__/__
	___X___X___ @__/__/__
	___X___X___ @__/__/__
3.	___X___X___ @__/__/__
	___X___X___ @__/__/__
	___X___X___ @__/__/__
	___X___X___ @__/__/__
	___X___X___ @__/__/__
4.	___X___X___ @__/__/__
	___X___X___ @__/__/__
	___X___X___ @__/__/__
	___X___X___ @__/__/__
	___X___X___ @__/__/__
5.	___X___X___ @__/__/__
	___X___X___ @__/__/__
	___X___X___ @__/__/__
	___X___X___ @__/__/__
	___X___X___ @__/__/__
6.	___X___X___ @__/__/__
	___X___X___ @__/__/__
	___X___X___ @__/__/__
	___X___X___ @__/__/__
	___X___X___ @__/__/__
7.	___X___X___ @__/__/__
	___X___X___ @__/__/__
	___X___X___ @__/__/__
	___X___X___ @__/__/__
	___X___X___ @__/__/__
8.	___X___X___ @__/__/__
	___X___X___ @__/__/__
	___X___X___ @__/__/__
	___X___X___ @__/__/__
	___X___X___ @__/__/__
9.	___X___X___ @__/__/__
	___X___X___ @__/__/__
	___X___X___ @__/__/__
	___X___X___ @__/__/__
	___X___X___ @__/__/__

2

CARDIO SESSION #1

TIME:_____

ACTIVITY:_____

DURATION:_____ LEVEL_____

DISTANCE:_____

CALORIES BURNED:_____

ACTIVITY PULSE RATE:_____bpm

RECOVERY PULSE RATE:_____bpm

DIFFERENCE:

DAILY SLEEP TRACKER

TIME TO BED:_____

TIME UP:_____

HOURS OF SLEEP:_____

COMMENTS:_____

DAILY AB TRACKER

EXERCISE	SET X REPS X WGT
1._____	___X___X___
2._____	___X___X___
3._____	___X___X___
4._____	___X___X___
5._____	___X___X___

FITNESS CLASS
(or any physical activity-walk, jog, squash)

START:_____ FINISH:_____

TYPE:_____

INSTRUCTOR:_____

ESTIMATE OF
CALORIES BURNED: [   ]

COMMENTS:_____

CARDIO SESSION #2

TIME:_____

ACTIVITY:_____

DURATION:_____ LEVEL_____

DISTANCE:_____

CALORIES BURNED:_____

ACTIVITY PULSE RATE:_____bpm

RECOVERY PULSE RATE:_____bpm

DIFFERENCE:_____

COMMENTS:_____

TOTAL CALORIES
BURNED TODAY: [   ]

NUTRITION			Points Goal	CAL *option*	PROT *grams*	FAT *grams*	CARB *grams*
Meal #1 – Time:	H₂O___Cups(L)						
Meal #2 – Time:	H₂O___Cups(L)						
Meal #3 – Time:	H₂O___Cups(L)						
Meal #4 – Time:	H₂O___Cups(L)						
Meal #5 – Time:	H₂O___Cups(L)						
Meal #6 – Time:	H₂O___Cups(L)						

2

Food Point Total For Today:					
Difference *(Goal Points Minus Actual Points)*					
Daily Totals: *(Add up each nutrient column. Convert each to calories. Add all and enter in "Total Calories")*		g	g	g	

Conversion To Calories Multiply Total Grams of **Pro X 4** = Calories Multiply Total Grams of **Carb X 4**=Calories Multiply Total Grams of **Fat X 9** = Calories	**Total Calories**	cal	cal	cal

Daily Percentages: *(Divide total calories of each nutrient by the Total Number of Calories)*	%	%	%

Total Calories Consumed:___

VS   **Difference**

Total Calories Burned: ___

Personal Training Log

WEIGHT TRAINING

Date:_____ Phase:_____

Start:_____ Finish:_____ Duration:_____

Day:_____ Warm Up:_____

EXERCISE	SET X REPS X WEIGHT @ TEMPO
1.	___X___X_____@__/__/__
	___X___X_____@__/__/__
	___X___X_____@__/__/__
	___X___X_____@__/__/__
	___X___X_____@__/__/__
2.	___X___X_____@__/__/__
	___X___X_____@__/__/__
	___X___X_____@__/__/__
	___X___X_____@__/__/__
	___X___X_____@__/__/__
3.	___X___X_____@__/__/__
	___X___X_____@__/__/__
	___X___X_____@__/__/__
	___X___X_____@__/__/__
	___X___X_____@__/__/__
4.	___X___X_____@__/__/__
	___X___X_____@__/__/__
	___X___X_____@__/__/__
	___X___X_____@__/__/__
	___X___X_____@__/__/__
5.	___X___X_____@__/__/__
	___X___X_____@__/__/__
	___X___X_____@__/__/__
	___X___X_____@__/__/__
	___X___X_____@__/__/__
6.	___X___X_____@__/__/__
	___X___X_____@__/__/__
	___X___X_____@__/__/__
	___X___X_____@__/__/__
	___X___X_____@__/__/__
7.	___X___X_____@__/__/__
	___X___X_____@__/__/__
	___X___X_____@__/__/__
	___X___X_____@__/__/__
	___X___X_____@__/__/__
8.	___X___X_____@__/__/__
	___X___X_____@__/__/__
	___X___X_____@__/__/__
	___X___X_____@__/__/__
	___X___X_____@__/__/__
9.	___X___X_____@__/__/__
	___X___X_____@__/__/__
	___X___X_____@__/__/__
	___X___X_____@__/__/__
	___X___X_____@__/__/__

CARDIO SESSION #1

TIME:_____

ACTIVITY:_____

DURATION:_____LEVEL_____

DISTANCE:_____

CALORIES BURNED:_____

ACTIVITY PULSE RATE:_____bpm

RECOVERY PULSE RATE:_____bpm

DIFFERENCE:

DAILY SLEEP TRACKER

TIME TO BED:_____

TIME UP:_____

HOURS OF SLEEP:_____

COMMENTS:_____

DAILY AB TRACKER

EXERCISE	SET X REPS X WGT
1._____	___X___X_____
2._____	___X___X_____
3._____	___X___X_____
4._____	___X___X_____
5._____	___X___X_____

FITNESS CLASS
(or any physical activity-walk, jog, squash)

START:_____FINISH:_____

TYPE:_____

INSTRUCTOR:_____

ESTIMATE OF
CALORIES BURNED:

COMMENTS:_____

CARDIO SESSION #2

TIME:_____

ACTIVITY:_____

DURATION:_____LEVEL_____

DISTANCE:_____

CALORIES BURNED:_____

ACTIVITY PULSE RATE:_____bpm

RECOVERY PULSE RATE:_____bpm

DIFFERENCE:_____

COMMENTS:_____

TOTAL CALORIES
BURNED TODAY:

Daily Nutrition Tracking

NUTRITION	Points Goal	CAL option	PROT grams	FAT grams	CARB grams
Meal #1 – Time: H₂O____Cups(L)					
Meal #2 – Time: H₂O____Cups(L)					
Meal #3 – Time: H₂O____Cups(L)					
Meal #4 – Time: H₂O____Cups(L)					
Meal #5 – Time: H₂O____Cups(L)					
Meal #6 – Time: H₂O____Cups(L)					
Food Point Total For Today:					
Difference (Goal Points Minus Actual Points)					
Daily Totals: (Add up each nutrient column. Convert each to calories. Add all and enter in "Total Calories")			g	g	g
Conversion To Calories Multiply Total Grams of **Pro X 4** = Calories / Multiply Total Grams of **Carb X 4**=Calories / Multiply Total Grams of **Fat X 9** = Calories	***Total Calories***		cal	cal	cal
Daily Percentages: (Divide total calories of each nutrient by the Total Number of Calories)			%	%	%

Total Calories Consumed:_____
VS   *Difference*
Total Calories Burned: _____

2

Personal Training Log

WEIGHT TRAINING

Date:_____ Phase:_____

Start:_____ Finish:_____ Duration:_____

Day:_____ Warm Up:_____

EXERCISE	SET X REPS X WEIGHT @ TEMPO
1.	___X___X___@__/__/__
	___X___X___@__/__/__
	___X___X___@__/__/__
	___X___X___@__/__/__
	___X___X___@__/__/__
2.	___X___X___@__/__/__
	___X___X___@__/__/__
	___X___X___@__/__/__
	___X___X___@__/__/__
	___X___X___@__/__/__
3.	___X___X___@__/__/__
	___X___X___@__/__/__
	___X___X___@__/__/__
	___X___X___@__/__/__
	___X___X___@__/__/__
4.	___X___X___@__/__/__
	___X___X___@__/__/__
	___X___X___@__/__/__
	___X___X___@__/__/__
	___X___X___@__/__/__
5.	___X___X___@__/__/__
	___X___X___@__/__/__
	___X___X___@__/__/__
	___X___X___@__/__/__
	___X___X___@__/__/__
6.	___X___X___@__/__/__
	___X___X___@__/__/__
	___X___X___@__/__/__
	___X___X___@__/__/__
	___X___X___@__/__/__
7.	___X___X___@__/__/__
	___X___X___@__/__/__
	___X___X___@__/__/__
	___X___X___@__/__/__
	___X___X___@__/__/__
8.	___X___X___@__/__/__
	___X___X___@__/__/__
	___X___X___@__/__/__
	___X___X___@__/__/__
	___X___X___@__/__/__
9.	___X___X___@__/__/__
	___X___X___@__/__/__
	___X___X___@__/__/__
	___X___X___@__/__/__
	___X___X___@__/__/__

CARDIO SESSION #1

TIME:_____

ACTIVITY:_____

DURATION:_____ LEVEL_____

DISTANCE:_____

CALORIES BURNED:_____

ACTIVITY PULSE RATE:_____bpm

RECOVERY PULSE RATE:_____bpm

DIFFERENCE:

DAILY SLEEP TRACKER

TIME TO BED:_____

TIME UP:_____

HOURS OF SLEEP:_____

COMMENTS:_____

DAILY AB TRACKER

EXERCISE	SET X REPS X WGT
1._____	___X___X___
2._____	___X___X___
3._____	___X___X___
4._____	___X___X___
5._____	___X___X___

FITNESS CLASS
(or any physical activity-walk, jog, squash)

START:_____ FINISH:_____

TYPE:_____

INSTRUCTOR:_____

ESTIMATE OF
CALORIES BURNED:

COMMENTS:_____

CARDIO SESSION #2

TIME:_____

ACTIVITY:_____

DURATION:_____ LEVEL_____

DISTANCE:_____

CALORIES BURNED:_____

ACTIVITY PULSE RATE:_____bpm

RECOVERY PULSE RATE:_____bpm

DIFFERENCE:_____

COMMENTS:_____

TOTAL CALORIES
BURNED TODAY:

NUTRITION	Points Goal	CAL *option*	PROT *grams*	FAT *grams*	CARB *grams*
Meal #1 – Time: H₂O____Cups(L)					
Meal #2 – Time: H₂O____Cups(L)					
Meal #3 – Time: H₂O____Cups(L)					
Meal #4 – Time: H₂O____Cups(L)					
Meal #5 – Time: H₂O____Cups(L)					
Meal #6 Time: H₂O____Cups(L)					
Food Point Total For Today:					
Difference (Goal Points Minus Actual Points)					
Daily Totals:(*Add up each nutrient column. Convert each to calories. Add all and enter in "Total Calories"*)			*g*	*g*	*g*
Conversion To Calories **Total** Multiply Total Grams of **Pro X 4** = Calories **Calories** Multiply Total Grams of **Carb X 4**=Calories Multiply Total Grams of **Fat X 9** = Calories			*cal*	*cal*	*cal*
Daily Percentages: (*Divide total calories of each nutrient by the Total Number of Calories*)			___ *%*	___ *%*	___ *%*

Total Calories Consumed:_____

                    VS   **Difference**

Total Calories Burned: _____

2

Personal Training Log

WEIGHT TRAINING

Date:_____ Phase:_____

Start:_____ Finish:_____ Duration:_____

Day:_____ Warm Up:_____

EXERCISE	SET X REPS X WEIGHT @ TEMPO
1.	___X___X_____@__/__/__
	___X___X_____@__/__/__
	___X___X_____@__/__/__
	___X___X_____@__/__/__
	___X___X_____@__/__/__
2.	___X___X_____@__/__/__
	___X___X_____@__/__/__
	___X___X_____@__/__/__
	___X___X_____@__/__/__
	___X___X_____@__/__/__
3.	___X___X_____@__/__/__
	___X___X_____@__/__/__
	___X___X_____@__/__/__
	___X___X_____@__/__/__
	___X___X_____@__/__/__
4.	___X___X_____@__/__/__
	___X___X_____@__/__/__
	___X___X_____@__/__/__
	___X___X_____@__/__/__
	___X___X_____@__/__/__
5.	___X___X_____@__/__/__
	___X___X_____@__/__/__
	___X___X_____@__/__/__
	___X___X_____@__/__/__
	___X___X_____@__/__/__
6.	___X___X_____@__/__/__
	___X___X_____@__/__/__
	___X___X_____@__/__/__
	___X___X_____@__/__/__
	___X___X_____@__/__/__
7.	___X___X_____@__/__/__
	___X___X_____@__/__/__
	___X___X_____@__/__/__
	___X___X_____@__/__/__
	___X___X_____@__/__/__
8.	___X___X_____@__/__/__
	___X___X_____@__/__/__
	___X___X_____@__/__/__
	___X___X_____@__/__/__
	___X___X_____@__/__/__
9.	___X___X_____@__/__/__
	___X___X_____@__/__/__
	___X___X_____@__/__/__
	___X___X_____@__/__/__
	___X___X_____@__/__/__

CARDIO SESSION #1

TIME:_____

ACTIVITY:_____

DURATION:_____ LEVEL_____

DISTANCE:_____

CALORIES BURNED:_____

ACTIVITY PULSE RATE:_____bpm

RECOVERY PULSE RATE:_____bpm

DIFFERENCE:

DAILY SLEEP TRACKER

TIME TO BED:_____

TIME UP:_____

HOURS OF SLEEP:_____

COMMENTS:_____

DAILY AB TRACKER

EXERCISE	SET X REPS X WGT
1._____	___X___X_____
2._____	___X___X_____
3._____	___X___X_____
4._____	___X___X_____
5._____	___X___X_____

FITNESS CLASS
(or any physical activity-walk, jog, squash)

START:_____ FINISH:_____

TYPE:_____

INSTRUCTOR:_____

ESTIMATE OF
CALORIES BURNED: [ ]

COMMENTS:_____

CARDIO SESSION #2

TIME:_____

ACTIVITY:_____

DURATION:_____ LEVEL_____

DISTANCE:_____

CALORIES BURNED:_____

ACTIVITY PULSE RATE:_____bpm

RECOVERY PULSE RATE:_____bpm

DIFFERENCE:_____

COMMENTS:_____

TOTAL CALORIES
BURNED TODAY: [ ]

NUTRITION	Points Goal	CAL *option*	PROT *grams*	FAT *grams*	CARB *grams*
Meal #1 – Time: H_2O_____Cups(L)					
Meal #2 – Time: H_2O_____Cups(L)					
Meal #3 – Time: H_2O_____Cups(L)					
Meal #4 – Time: H_2O_____Cups(L)					
Meal #5 – Time: H_2O_____Cups(L)					
Meal #6 – Time: H_2O_____Cups(L)					
Food Point Total For Today:					
Difference (Goal Points Minus Actual Points)					
Daily Totals: *(Add up each nutrient column. Convert each to calories. Add all and enter in "Total Calories")*			g	g	g
Conversion To Calories *Multiply Total Grams of **Pro X 4** = Calories* *Multiply Total Grams of **Carb X 4**=Calories* *Multiply Total Grams of **Fat X 9** = Calories*	**Total Calories**		cal	cal	cal
Daily Percentages: *(Divide total calories of each nutrient by the Total Number of Calories)*			___ %	___ %	___ %

2

Total Calories Consumed:_____

VS   **Difference**

Total Calories Burned: _____

Personal Training Log

WEIGHT TRAINING

Date:_____ Phase:_____

Start:_____ Finish:_____ Duration:_____

Day:_____ Warm Up:_____

EXERCISE	SET X REPS X WEIGHT @ TEMPO
1.	__X__X_____@__/__/__
	__X__X_____@__/__/__
	__X__X_____@__/__/__
	__X__X_____@__/__/__
	__X__X_____@__/__/__
2.	__X__X_____@__/__/__
	__X__X_____@__/__/__
	__X__X_____@__/__/__
	__X__X_____@__/__/__
	__X__X_____@__/__/__
3.	__X__X_____@__/__/__
	__X__X_____@__/__/__
	__X__X_____@__/__/__
	__X__X_____@__/__/__
	__X__X_____@__/__/__
4.	__X__X_____@__/__/__
	__X__X_____@__/__/__
	__X__X_____@__/__/__
	__X__X_____@__/__/__
	__X__X_____@__/__/__
5.	__X__X_____@__/__/__
	__X__X_____@__/__/__
	__X__X_____@__/__/__
	__X__X_____@__/__/__
	__X__X_____@__/__/__
6.	__X__X_____@__/__/__
	__X__X_____@__/__/__
	__X__X_____@__/__/__
	__X__X_____@__/__/__
	__X__X_____@__/__/__
7.	__X__X_____@__/__/__
	__X__X_____@__/__/__
	__X__X_____@__/__/__
	__X__X_____@__/__/__
8.	__X__X_____@__/__/__
	__X__X_____@__/__/__
	__X__X_____@__/__/__
	__X__X_____@__/__/__
	__X__X_____@__/__/__
9.	__X__X_____@__/__/__
	__X__X_____@__/__/__
	__X__X_____@__/__/__
	__X__X_____@__/__/__
	__X__X_____@__/__/__

CARDIO SESSION #1

TIME:_____

ACTIVITY:_____

DURATION:_____ LEVEL_____

DISTANCE:_____

CALORIES BURNED:_____

ACTIVITY PULSE RATE:_____ bpm

RECOVERY PULSE RATE:_____ bpm

DIFFERENCE:

DAILY SLEEP TRACKER

TIME TO BED:_____

TIME UP:_____

HOURS OF SLEEP:_____

COMMENTS:_____

DAILY AB TRACKER

EXERCISE	SET X REPS X WGT
1._____	__X__X___
2._____	__X__X___
3._____	__X__X___
4._____	__X__X___
5._____	__X__X___

FITNESS CLASS
(or any physical activity-walk, jog, squash)

START:_____ FINISH:_____

TYPE:_____

INSTRUCTOR:_____

ESTIMATE OF
CALORIES BURNED:

COMMENTS:_____

CARDIO SESSION #2

TIME:_____

ACTIVITY:_____

DURATION:_____ LEVEL_____

DISTANCE:_____

CALORIES BURNED:_____

ACTIVITY PULSE RATE:_____ bpm

RECOVERY PULSE RATE:_____ bpm

DIFFERENCE:_____

COMMENTS:_____

TOTAL CALORIES
BURNED TODAY:

NUTRITION	Points Goal	CAL *option*	PROT *grams*	FAT *grams*	CARB *grams*
Meal #1 – Time:　　　H₂O___Cups(L)					
Meal #2 – Time:　　　H₂O___Cups(L)					
Meal #3 – Time:　　　H₂O___Cups(L)					
Meal #4 – Time:　　　H₂O___Cups(L)					
Meal #5 – Time:　　　H₂O___Cups(L)					
Meal #6 – Time:　　　H₂O___Cups(L)					
Food Point Total For Today:					
Difference (Goal Points Minus Actual Points)					
Daily Totals: *(Add up each nutrient column. Convert each to calories. Add all and enter in "Total Calories")*			g	g	g
Conversion To Calories Multiply Total Grams of **Pro X 4** = Calories Multiply Total Grams of **Carb X 4**=Calories Multiply Total Grams of **Fat X 9** = Calories	**Total Calories**		cal	cal	cal
Daily Percentages: (Divide total calories of each nutrient by the Total Number of Calories)			%	%	%

Total Calories Consumed:_____
VS　　　　　　　　**Difference**
Total Calories Burned: _____

Personal Training Log

WEIGHT TRAINING

Date:_____ Phase:_____

Start:_____ Finish:_____ Duration:_____

Day:_____ Warm Up:_____

EXERCISE	SET X REPS X WEIGHT @ TEMPO
1.	___ X ___ X _____ @__/__/__
	___ X ___ X _____ @__/__/__
	___ X ___ X _____ @__/__/__
	___ X ___ X _____ @__/__/__
	___ X ___ X _____ @__/__/__
2.	___ X ___ X _____ @__/__/__
	___ X ___ X _____ @__/__/__
	___ X ___ X _____ @__/__/__
	___ X ___ X _____ @__/__/__
	___ X ___ X _____ @__/__/__
3.	___ X ___ X _____ @__/__/__
	___ X ___ X _____ @__/__/__
	___ X ___ X _____ @__/__/__
	___ X ___ X _____ @__/__/__
	___ X ___ X _____ @__/__/__
4.	___ X ___ X _____ @__/__/__
	___ X ___ X _____ @__/__/__
	___ X ___ X _____ @__/__/__
	___ X ___ X _____ @__/__/__
	___ X ___ X _____ @__/__/__
5.	___ X ___ X _____ @__/__/__
	___ X ___ X _____ @__/__/__
	___ X ___ X _____ @__/__/__
	___ X ___ X _____ @__/__/__
	___ X ___ X _____ @__/__/__
6.	___ X ___ X _____ @__/__/__
	___ X ___ X _____ @__/__/__
	___ X ___ X _____ @__/__/__
	___ X ___ X _____ @__/__/__
	___ X ___ X _____ @__/__/__
7.	___ X ___ X _____ @__/__/__
	___ X ___ X _____ @__/__/__
	___ X ___ X _____ @__/__/__
	___ X ___ X _____ @__/__/__
	___ X ___ X _____ @__/__/__
8.	___ X ___ X _____ @__/__/__
	___ X ___ X _____ @__/__/__
	___ X ___ X _____ @__/__/__
	___ X ___ X _____ @__/__/__
	___ X ___ X _____ @__/__/__
9.	___ X ___ X _____ @__/__/__
	___ X ___ X _____ @__/__/__
	___ X ___ X _____ @__/__/__
	___ X ___ X _____ @__/__/__
	___ X ___ X _____ @__/__/__

CARDIO SESSION #1

TIME:_____

ACTIVITY:_____

DURATION:_____LEVEL_____

DISTANCE:_____

CALORIES BURNED:_____

ACTIVITY PULSE RATE:_____bpm

RECOVERY PULSE RATE:_____bpm

DIFFERENCE:_____

DAILY SLEEP TRACKER

TIME TO BED:_____

TIME UP:_____

HOURS OF SLEEP:_____

COMMENTS:_____

DAILY AB TRACKER

EXERCISE	SET X REPS X WGT
1._____	___ X ___ X_____
2._____	___ X ___ X_____
3._____	___ X ___ X_____
4._____	___ X ___ X_____
5._____	___ X ___ X_____

FITNESS CLASS
(or any physical activity-walk, jog, squash)

START:_____FINISH:_____

TYPE:_____

INSTRUCTOR:_____

ESTIMATE OF
CALORIES BURNED:

COMMENTS:_____

CARDIO SESSION #2

TIME:_____

ACTIVITY:_____

DURATION:_____LEVEL_____

DISTANCE:_____

CALORIES BURNED:_____

ACTIVITY PULSE RATE:_____bpm

RECOVERY PULSE RATE:_____bpm

DIFFERENCE:_____

COMMENTS:_____

_____

TOTAL CALORIES
BURNED TODAY:

NUTRITION	Points Goal	CAL option	PROT grams	FAT grams	CARB grams
Meal #1 – Time: H₂O_____Cups(L)					
Meal #2 – Time: H₂O_____Cups(L)					
Meal #3 – Time: H₂O_____Cups(L)					
Meal #4 – Time: H₂O_____Cups(L)					
Meal #5 – Time: H₂O_____Cups(L)					
Meal #6 – Time: H₂O_____Cups(L)					
Food Point Total For Today:					
Difference (Goal Points Minus Actual Points)					
Daily Totals: (Add up each nutrient column. Convert each to calories. Add all and enter in "Total Calories")			*g*	*g*	*g*
Conversion To Calories Multiply Total Grams of **Pro X 4** = Calories Multiply Total Grams of **Carb X 4** = Calories Multiply Total Grams of **Fat X 9** = Calories	**Total Calories**		*cal*	*cal*	*cal*
Daily Percentages: (Divide total calories of each nutrient by the Total Number of Calories)			___ %	___ %	___ %
Total Calories Consumed:_____ VS **Total Calories Burned:** _____	**Difference**				

2

Personal Training Log

WEIGHT TRAINING

Date:_____ Phase:_____

Start:_____ Finish:_____ Duration:_____

Day:_____ Warm Up:_____

EXERCISE	SET X REPS X WEIGHT @ TEMPO
1.	___X___X_____@__/__/__
	___X___X_____@__/__/__
	___X___X_____@__/__/__
	___X___X_____@__/__/__
	___X___X_____@__/__/__
2.	___X___X_____@__/__/__
	___X___X_____@__/__/__
	___X___X_____@__/__/__
	___X___X_____@__/__/__
	___X___X_____@__/__/__
3.	___X___X_____@__/__/__
	___X___X_____@__/__/__
	___X___X_____@__/__/__
	___X___X_____@__/__/__
	___X___X_____@__/__/__
4.	___X___X_____@__/__/__
	___X___X_____@__/__/__
	___X___X_____@__/__/__
	___X___X_____@__/__/__
	___X___X_____@__/__/__
5.	___X___X_____@__/__/__
	___X___X_____@__/__/__
	___X___X_____@__/__/__
	___X___X_____@__/__/__
	___X___X_____@__/__/__
6.	___X___X_____@__/__/__
	___X___X_____@__/__/__
	___X___X_____@__/__/__
	___X___X_____@__/__/__
	___X___X_____@__/__/__
7.	___X___X_____@__/__/__
	___X___X_____@__/__/__
	___X___X_____@__/__/__
	___X___X_____@__/__/__
	___X___X_____@__/__/__
8.	___X___X_____@__/__/__
	___X___X_____@__/__/__
	___X___X_____@__/__/__
	___X___X_____@__/__/__
	___X___X_____@__/__/__
9.	___X___X_____@__/__/__
	___X___X_____@__/__/__
	___X___X_____@__/__/__
	___X___X_____@__/__/__
	___X___X_____@__/__/__

CARDIO SESSION #1

TIME:_____

ACTIVITY:_____

DURATION:_____ LEVEL_____

DISTANCE:_____

CALORIES BURNED:_____

ACTIVITY PULSE RATE:_____ bpm

RECOVERY PULSE RATE:_____ bpm

DIFFERENCE:

DAILY SLEEP TRACKER

TIME TO BED:_____

TIME UP:_____

HOURS OF SLEEP:_____

COMMENTS:_____

DAILY AB TRACKER

EXERCISE	SET X REPS X WGT
1._____	___X___X____
2._____	___X___X____
3._____	___X___X____
4._____	___X___X____
5._____	___X___X____

FITNESS CLASS

(or any physical activity-walk, jog, squash)

START:_____ FINISH:_____

TYPE:_____

INSTRUCTOR:_____

ESTIMATE OF
CALORIES BURNED: [   ]

COMMENTS:_____

CARDIO SESSION #2

TIME:_____

ACTIVITY:_____

DURATION:_____ LEVEL_____

DISTANCE:_____

CALORIES BURNED:_____

ACTIVITY PULSE RATE:_____ bpm

RECOVERY PULSE RATE:_____ bpm

DIFFERENCE:_____

COMMENTS:_____

_____

TOTAL CALORIES
BURNED TODAY: [   ]

NUTRITION	Points Goal	CAL *option*	PROT *grams*	FAT *grams*	CARB *grams*
Meal #1 – Time: H₂O____Cups(L)					
Meal #2 – Time: H₂O____Cups(L)					
Meal #3 – Time: H₂O____Cups(L)					
Meal #4 – Time: H₂O____Cups(L)					
Meal #5 – Time: H₂O____Cups(L)					
Meal #6 – Time: H₂O____Cups(L)					

2

	Points				
Food Point Total For Today:					
Difference (Goal Points Minus Actual Points)					
Daily Totals: *(Add up each nutrient column. Convert each to calories. Add all and enter in "Total Calories")*			g	g	g
Conversion To Calories Multiply Total Grams of *Pro X 4* = Calories; Multiply Total Grams of *Carb X 4*=Calories; Multiply Total Grams of *Fat X 9* = Calories	**Total Calories**		cal	cal	cal
Daily Percentages: (Divide total calories of each nutrient by the Total Number of Calories)			___%	___%	___%

Total Calories Consumed:_____
VS   **Difference**
Total Calories Burned: _____

Personal Training Log

WEIGHT TRAINING

Date:_____ Phase:_____

Start:_____ Finish:_____ Duration:_____

Day:_____ Warm Up:_____

EXERCISE	SET X REPS X WEIGHT @ TEMPO
1.	___ X ___ X _____ @___/__/___
	___ X ___ X _____ @___/__/___
	___ X ___ X _____ @___/__/___
	___ X ___ X _____ @___/__/___
	___ X ___ X _____ @___/__/___
2.	___ X ___ X _____ @___/__/___
	___ X ___ X _____ @___/__/___
	___ X ___ X _____ @___/__/___
	___ X ___ X _____ @___/__/___
	___ X ___ X _____ @___/__/___
3.	___ X ___ X _____ @___/__/___
	___ X ___ X _____ @___/__/___
	___ X ___ X _____ @___/__/___
	___ X ___ X _____ @___/__/___
	___ X ___ X _____ @___/__/___
4.	___ X ___ X _____ @___/__/___
	___ X ___ X _____ @___/__/___
	___ X ___ X _____ @___/__/___
	___ X ___ X _____ @___/__/___
	___ X ___ X _____ @___/__/___
5.	___ X ___ X _____ @___/__/___
	___ X ___ X _____ @___/__/___
	___ X ___ X _____ @___/__/___
	___ X ___ X _____ @___/__/___
	___ X ___ X _____ @___/__/___
6.	___ X ___ X _____ @___/__/___
	___ X ___ X _____ @___/__/___
	___ X ___ X _____ @___/__/___
	___ X ___ X _____ @___/__/___
	___ X ___ X _____ @___/__/___
7.	___ X ___ X _____ @___/__/___
	___ X ___ X _____ @___/__/___
	___ X ___ X _____ @___/__/___
	___ X ___ X _____ @___/__/___
	___ X ___ X _____ @___/__/___
8.	___ X ___ X _____ @___/__/___
	___ X ___ X _____ @___/__/___
	___ X ___ X _____ @___/__/___
	___ X ___ X _____ @___/__/___
	___ X ___ X _____ @___/__/___
9.	___ X ___ X _____ @___/__/___
	___ X ___ X _____ @___/__/___
	___ X ___ X _____ @___/__/___
	___ X ___ X _____ @___/__/___
	___ X ___ X _____ @___/__/___

CARDIO SESSION #1

TIME:_____

ACTIVITY:_____

DURATION:_____ LEVEL_____

DISTANCE:_____

CALORIES BURNED:_____

ACTIVITY PULSE RATE:_____bpm

RECOVERY PULSE RATE:_____bpm

DIFFERENCE:_____

DAILY SLEEP TRACKER

TIME TO BED:_____

TIME UP:_____

HOURS OF SLEEP:_____

COMMENTS:_____

DAILY AB TRACKER

EXERCISE	SET X REPS X WGT
1._____	___X___X_____
2._____	___X___X_____
3._____	___X___X_____
4._____	___X___X_____
5._____	___X___X_____

FITNESS CLASS
(or any physical activity-walk, jog, squash)

START:_____ FINISH:_____

TYPE:_____

INSTRUCTOR:_____

ESTIMATE OF
CALORIES BURNED: [   ]

COMMENTS:_____

CARDIO SESSION #2

TIME:_____

ACTIVITY:_____

DURATION:_____ LEVEL_____

DISTANCE:_____

CALORIES BURNED:_____

ACTIVITY PULSE RATE:_____bpm

RECOVERY PULSE RATE:_____bpm

DIFFERENCE:_____

COMMENTS:_____

TOTAL CALORIES
BURNED TODAY: [   ]

NUTRITION	Points Goal	CAL *option*	PROT *grams*	FAT *grams*	CARB *grams*
Meal #1 – Time: H₂O_____Cups(L)					
Meal #2 – Time: H₂O_____Cups(L)					
Meal #3 – Time: H₂O_____Cups(L)					
Meal #4 – Time: H₂O_____Cups(L)					
Meal #5 – Time: H₂O_____Cups(L)					
Meal #6 – Time: H₂O_____Cups(L)					
Food Point Total For Today:					
Difference (Goal Points Minus Actual Points)					
Daily Totals: *(Add up each nutrient column. Convert each to calories. Add all and enter in "Total Calories")*			*g*	*g*	*g*
Conversion To Calories Multiply Total Grams of **Pro X 4** = Calories Multiply Total Grams of **Carb X 4** =Calories Multiply Total Grams of **Fat X 9** = Calories	*Total Calories*		*cal*	*cal*	*cal*
Daily Percentages: (Divide total calories of each nutrient by the Total Number of Calories)			___ %	___ %	___ %

Total Calories Consumed:_____
               VS   ***Difference***
Total Calories Burned: _____

2

Personal Training Log

WEIGHT TRAINING

Date:_____ Phase:_____

Start:_____ Finish:_____ Duration:_____

Day:_____ Warm Up:_____

EXERCISE	SET X REPS X WEIGHT @ TEMPO
1.	____X____X_____@__/__/__
	____X____X_____@__/__/__
	____X____X_____@__/__/__
	____X____X_____@__/__/__
	____X____X_____@__/__/__
2.	____X____X_____@__/__/__
	____X____X_____@__/__/__
	____X____X_____@__/__/__
	____X____X_____@__/__/__
	____X____X_____@__/__/__
3.	____X____X_____@__/__/__
	____X____X_____@__/__/__
	____X____X_____@__/__/__
	____X____X_____@__/__/__
	____X____X_____@__/__/__
4.	____X____X_____@__/__/__
	____X____X_____@__/__/__
	____X____X_____@__/__/__
	____X____X_____@__/__/__
	____X____X_____@__/__/__
5.	____X____X_____@__/__/__
	____X____X_____@__/__/__
	____X____X_____@__/__/__
	____X____X_____@__/__/__
	____X____X_____@__/__/__
6.	____X____X_____@__/__/__
	____X____X_____@__/__/__
	____X____X_____@__/__/__
	____X____X_____@__/__/__
	____X____X_____@__/__/__
7.	____X____X_____@__/__/__
	____X____X_____@__/__/__
	____X____X_____@__/__/__
	____X____X_____@__/__/__
	____X____X_____@__/__/__
8.	____X____X_____@__/__/__
	____X____X_____@__/__/__
	____X____X_____@__/__/__
	____X____X_____@__/__/__
	____X____X_____@__/__/__
9.	____X____X_____@__/__/__
	____X____X_____@__/__/__
	____X____X_____@__/__/__
	____X____X_____@__/__/__
	____X____X_____@__/__/__

CARDIO SESSION #1

TIME:_____

ACTIVITY:_____

DURATION:_____ LEVEL_____

DISTANCE:_____

CALORIES BURNED:_____

ACTIVITY PULSE RATE:_____bpm

RECOVERY PULSE RATE:_____bpm

DIFFERENCE:

DAILY SLEEP TRACKER

TIME TO BED:_____

TIME UP:_____

HOURS OF SLEEP:_____

COMMENTS:_____

DAILY AB TRACKER

EXERCISE	SET X REPS X WGT
1._____	____X____X_____
2._____	____X____X_____
3._____	____X____X_____
4._____	____X____X_____
5._____	____X____X_____

FITNESS CLASS
(or any physical activity-walk, jog, squash)

START:_____ FINISH:_____

TYPE:_____

INSTRUCTOR:_____

ESTIMATE OF
CALORIES BURNED:

COMMENTS:_____

CARDIO SESSION #2

TIME:_____

ACTIVITY:_____

DURATION:_____ LEVEL_____

DISTANCE:_____

CALORIES BURNED:_____

ACTIVITY PULSE RATE:_____bpm

RECOVERY PULSE RATE:_____bpm

DIFFERENCE:_____

COMMENTS:_____

TOTAL CALORIES
BURNED TODAY:

2

NUTRITION		Points Goal	CAL *option*	PROT *grams*	FAT *grams*	CARB *grams*
Meal #1 – Time:	H$_2$O____Cups(L)					
Meal #2 – Time:	H$_2$O____Cups(L)					
Meal #3 – Time:	H$_2$O____Cups(L)					
Meal #4 – Time:	H$_2$O____Cups(L)					
Meal #5 – Time:	H$_2$O____Cups(L)					
Meal #6 – Time:	H$_2$O____Cups(L)					
Food Point Total For Today:						
Difference *(Goal Points Minus Actual Points)*						
Daily Totals: *(Add up each nutrient column. Convert each to calories. Add all and enter in "Total Calories")*				g	g	g
Conversion To Calories Multiply Total Grams of **Pro X 4** = Calories Multiply Total Grams of **Carb X 4**=Calories Multiply Total Grams of **Fat X 9** = Calories	**Total Calories**			cal	cal	cal
Daily Percentages: *(Divide total calories of each nutrient by the Total Number of Calories)*				%	%	%

Total Calories Consumed:_____
VS   *Difference*
Total Calories Burned: _____

Personal Training Log

WEIGHT TRAINING

Date:_____Phase:_____

Start:_____Finish:_____Duration:_____

Day:_____Warm Up:_____

EXERCISE	SET X REPS X WEIGHT @ TEMPO
1.	____X____X_____@__/__/__
	____X____X_____@__/__/__
	____X____X_____@__/__/__
	____X____X_____@__/__/__
	____X____X_____@__/__/__
2.	____X____X_____@__/__/__
	____X____X_____@__/__/__
	____X____X_____@__/__/__
	____X____X_____@__/__/__
	____X____X_____@__/__/__
3.	____X____X_____@__/__/__
	____X____X_____@__/__/__
	____X____X_____@__/__/__
	____X____X_____@__/__/__
	____X____X_____@__/__/__
4.	____X____X_____@__/__/__
	____X____X_____@__/__/__
	____X____X_____@__/__/__
	____X____X_____@__/__/__
	____X____X_____@__/__/__
5.	____X____X_____@__/__/__
	____X____X_____@__/__/__
	____X____X_____@__/__/__
	____X____X_____@__/__/__
	____X____X_____@__/__/__
6.	____X____X_____@__/__/__
	____X____X_____@__/__/__
	____X____X_____@__/__/__
	____X____X_____@__/__/__
	____X____X_____@__/__/__
7.	____X____X_____@__/__/__
	____X____X_____@__/__/__
	____X____X_____@__/__/__
	____X____X_____@__/__/__
	____X____X_____@__/__/__
8.	____X____X_____@__/__/__
	____X____X_____@__/__/__
	____X____X_____@__/__/__
	____X____X_____@__/__/__
	____X____X_____@__/__/__
9.	____X____X_____@__/__/__
	____X____X_____@__/__/__
	____X____X_____@__/__/__
	____X____X_____@__/__/__
	____X____X_____@__/__/__

CARDIO SESSION #1

TIME:_____

ACTIVITY:_____

DURATION:_____LEVEL_____

DISTANCE:_____

CALORIES BURNED:_____

ACTIVITY PULSE RATE:_____bpm

RECOVERY PULSE RATE:_____bpm

DIFFERENCE:

DAILY SLEEP TRACKER

TIME TO BED:_____

TIME UP:_____

HOURS OF SLEEP:_____

COMMENTS:_____

DAILY AB TRACKER

EXERCISE	SET X REPS X WGT
1._____	____X____X_____
2._____	____X____X_____
3._____	____X____X_____
4._____	____X____X_____
5._____	____X____X_____

FITNESS CLASS

(or any physical activity-walk, jog, squash)

START:_____FINISH:_____

TYPE:_____

INSTRUCTOR:_____

ESTIMATE OF
CALORIES BURNED:

COMMENTS:_____

CARDIO SESSION #2

TIME:_____

ACTIVITY:_____

DURATION:_____LEVEL_____

DISTANCE:_____

CALORIES BURNED:_____

ACTIVITY PULSE RATE:_____bpm

RECOVERY PULSE RATE:_____bpm

DIFFERENCE:_____

COMMENTS:_____

TOTAL CALORIES
BURNED TODAY:

NUTRITION		Points Goal	CAL *option*	PROT *grams*	FAT *grams*	CARB *grams*
Meal #1 – Time:	H$_2$O_____Cups(L)					
Meal #2 – Time:	H$_2$O_____Cups(L)					
Meal #3 – Time:	H$_2$O_____Cups(L)					
Meal #4 – Time:	H$_2$O_____Cups(L)					
Meal #5 – Time:	H$_2$O_____Cups(L)					
Meal #6 – Time:	H$_2$O_____Cups(L)					

Food Point Total For Today:		
Difference (Goal Points Minus Actual Points)		
Daily Totals: *(Add up each nutrient column. Convert each to calories. Add all and enter in "Total Calories")*		*g* *g* *g*
Conversion To Calories Multiply Total Grams of **Pro X 4** = Calories Multiply Total Grams of **Carb X 4**=Calories Multiply Total Grams of **Fat X 9** = Calories	**Total Calories**	*cal* *cal* *cal*
Daily Percentages: (Divide total calories of each nutrient by the Total Number of Calories)		___% ___% ___%

Total Calories Consumed:_____

      VS   *Difference*

Total Calories Burned: _____

2

Personal Training Log

WEIGHT TRAINING

Date:_____ Phase:_____

Start:_____ Finish:_____ Duration:_____

Day:_____ Warm Up:_____

EXERCISE	SET X REPS X WEIGHT @ TEMPO
1.	___X___X ___ @__/__/__
	___X___X ___ @__/__/__
	___X___X ___ @__/__/__
	___X___X ___ @__/__/__
	___X___X ___ @__/__/__
2.	___X___X ___ @__/__/__
	___X___X ___ @__/__/__
	___X___X ___ @__/__/__
	___X___X ___ @__/__/__
	___X___X ___ @__/__/__
3.	___X___X ___ @__/__/__
	___X___X ___ @__/__/__
	___X___X ___ @__/__/__
	___X___X ___ @__/__/__
	___X___X ___ @__/__/__
4.	___X___X ___ @__/__/__
	___X___X ___ @__/__/__
	___X___X ___ @__/__/__
	___X___X ___ @__/__/__
	___X___X ___ @__/__/__
5.	___X___X ___ @__/__/__
	___X___X ___ @__/__/__
	___X___X ___ @__/__/__
	___X___X ___ @__/__/__
	___X___X ___ @__/__/__
6.	___X___X ___ @__/__/__
	___X___X ___ @__/__/__
	___X___X ___ @__/__/__
	___X___X ___ @__/__/__
	___X___X ___ @__/__/__
7.	___X___X ___ @__/__/__
	___X___X ___ @__/__/__
	___X___X ___ @__/__/__
	___X___X ___ @__/__/__
	___X___X ___ @__/__/__
8.	___X___X ___ @__/__/__
	___X___X ___ @__/__/__
	___X___X ___ @__/__/__
	___X___X ___ @__/__/__
	___X___X ___ @__/__/__
9.	___X___X ___ @__/__/__
	___X___X ___ @__/__/__
	___X___X ___ @__/__/__
	___X___X ___ @__/__/__
	___X___X ___ @__/__/__

CARDIO SESSION #1

TIME:_____

ACTIVITY:_____

DURATION:_____ LEVEL_____

DISTANCE:_____

CALORIES BURNED:_____

ACTIVITY PULSE RATE:_____bpm

RECOVERY PULSE RATE:_____bpm

DIFFERENCE:

DAILY SLEEP TRACKER

TIME TO BED:_____

TIME UP:_____

HOURS OF SLEEP:_____

COMMENTS:_____

DAILY AB TRACKER

EXERCISE	SET X REPS X WGT
1._____	___X___X_____
2._____	___X___X_____
3._____	___X___X_____
4._____	___X___X_____
5._____	___X___X_____

FITNESS CLASS
(or any physical activity-walk, jog, squash)

START:_____ FINISH:_____

TYPE:_____

INSTRUCTOR:_____

ESTIMATE OF
CALORIES BURNED:

COMMENTS:_____

CARDIO SESSION #2

TIME:_____

ACTIVITY:_____

DURATION:_____ LEVEL_____

DISTANCE:_____

CALORIES BURNED:_____

ACTIVITY PULSE RATE:_____bpm

RECOVERY PULSE RATE:_____bpm

DIFFERENCE:_____

COMMENTS:_____

TOTAL CALORIES
BURNED TODAY:

Daily Nutrition Tracking

NUTRITION	Points Goal	CAL *option*	PROT *grams*	FAT *grams*	CARB *grams*
Meal #1 – Time: H₂O____Cups(L)					
Meal #2 – Time: H₂O____Cups(L)					
Meal #3 – Time: H₂O____Cups(L)					
Meal #4 – Time: H₂O____Cups(L)					
Meal #5 – Time: H₂O____Cups(L)					
Meal #6 – Time: H₂O____Cups(L)					

2

Food Point Total For Today:		
Difference (Goal Points Minus Actual Points)		

Daily Totals: *(Add up each nutrient column. Convert each to calories. Add all and enter in "Total Calories")* — g   g   g

Conversion To Calories
Multiply Total Grams of **Pro X 4** = Calories
Multiply Total Grams of **Carb X 4** = Calories
Multiply Total Grams of **Fat X 9** = Calories

Total Calories — cal   cal   cal

Daily Percentages: *(Divide total calories of each nutrient by the Total Number of Calories)* — %   %   %

Total Calories Consumed:_____
VS   **Difference**
Total Calories Burned: _____

Personal Training Log

2

WEIGHT TRAINING

Date:_____ Phase:_____

Start:_____ Finish:_____ Duration:_____

Day:_____ Warm Up:_____

EXERCISE	SET X REPS X WEIGHT @ TEMPO
1.	___X_____X_____@__/__/__
	___X_____X_____@__/__/__
	___X_____X_____@__/__/__
	___X_____X_____@__/__/__
	___X_____X_____@__/__/__
2.	___X_____X_____@__/__/__
	___X_____X_____@__/__/__
	___X_____X_____@__/__/__
	___X_____X_____@__/__/__
	___X_____X_____@__/__/__
3.	___X_____X_____@__/__/__
	___X_____X_____@__/__/__
	___X_____X_____@__/__/__
	___X_____X_____@__/__/__
	___X_____X_____@__/__/__
4.	___X_____X_____@__/__/__
	___X_____X_____@__/__/__
	___X_____X_____@__/__/__
	___X_____X_____@__/__/__
	___X_____X_____@__/__/__
5.	___X_____X_____@__/__/__
	___X_____X_____@__/__/__
	___X_____X_____@__/__/__
	___X_____X_____@__/__/__
	___X_____X_____@__/__/__
6.	___X_____X_____@__/__/__
	___X_____X_____@__/__/__
	___X_____X_____@__/__/__
	___X_____X_____@__/__/__
	___X_____X_____@__/__/__
7.	___X_____X_____@__/__/__
	___X_____X_____@__/__/__
	___X_____X_____@__/__/__
	___X_____X_____@__/__/__
	___X_____X_____@__/__/__
8.	___X_____X_____@__/__/__
	___X_____X_____@__/__/__
	___X_____X_____@__/__/__
	___X_____X_____@__/__/__
	___X_____X_____@__/__/__
9.	___X_____X_____@__/__/__
	___X_____X_____@__/__/__
	___X_____X_____@__/__/__
	___X_____X_____@__/__/__
	___X_____X_____@__/__/__

CARDIO SESSION #1

TIME:_____

ACTIVITY:_____

DURATION:_____LEVEL_____

DISTANCE:_____

CALORIES BURNED:_____

ACTIVITY PULSE RATE:_____bpm

RECOVERY PULSE RATE:_____bpm

DIFFERENCE:

DAILY SLEEP TRACKER

TIME TO BED:_____

TIME UP:_____

HOURS OF SLEEP:_____

COMMENTS:_____

DAILY AB TRACKER

EXERCISE	SET X REPS X WGT
1._____	___X_____X
2._____	___X_____X
3._____	___X_____X
4._____	___X_____X
5._____	___X_____X

FITNESS CLASS

(or any physical activity-walk, jog, squash)

START:_____FINISH:_____

TYPE:_____

INSTRUCTOR:_____

ESTIMATE OF
CALORIES BURNED: [   ]

COMMENTS:_____

CARDIO SESSION #2

TIME:_____

ACTIVITY:_____

DURATION:_____LEVEL_____

DISTANCE:_____

CALORIES BURNED:_____

ACTIVITY PULSE RATE:_____bpm

RECOVERY PULSE RATE:_____bpm

DIFFERENCE:_____

COMMENTS:_____

_____

TOTAL CALORIES
BURNED TODAY: [   ]

NUTRITION	Points Goal	CAL *option*	PROT *grams*	FAT *grams*	CARB *grams*
Meal #1 – Time:　　　　H₂O____Cups(L)					
Meal #2 – Time:　　　　H₂O____Cups(L)					
Meal #3 – Time:　　　　H₂O____Cups(L)					
Meal #4 – Time:　　　　H₂O____Cups(L)					
Meal #5 – Time:　　　　H₂O____Cups(L)					
Meal #6　Time:　　　　H₂O____Cups(L)					

Food Point Total For Today:					
Difference (Goal Points Minus Actual Points)					

Daily Totals: *(Add up each nutrient column. Convert each to calories. Add all and enter in "Total Calories")* 　　g　　g　　g

Conversion To Calories
Multiply Total Grams of **Pro X 4** = Calories
Multiply Total Grams of **Carb X 4**=Calories
Multiply Total Grams of **Fat X 9** = Calories

Total Calories　　　　cal　　cal　　cal

Daily Percentages: (Divide total calories of each nutrient by the Total Number of Calories)　　___%　___%　___%

Total Calories Consumed:_____
VS　　　　　　　　**Difference**
Total Calories Burned:　_____

Personal Training Log

WEIGHT TRAINING					CARDIO SESSION #1

WEIGHT TRAINING

Date:_____Phase:_____

Start:_____Finish:_____Duration:_____

Day:_____Warm Up:_____

EXERCISE	SET X REPS X WEIGHT @ TEMPO
1.	___X___X_____@__/__/__
	___X___X_____@__/__/__
	___X___X_____@__/__/__
	___X___X_____@__/__/__
	___X___X_____@__/__/__
2.	___X___X_____@__/__/__
	___X___X_____@__/__/__
	___X___X_____@__/__/__
	___X___X_____@__/__/__
	___X___X_____@__/__/__
3.	___X___X_____@__/__/__
	___X___X_____@__/__/__
	___X___X_____@__/__/__
	___X___X_____@__/__/__
	___X___X_____@__/__/__
4.	___X___X_____@__/__/__
	___X___X_____@__/__/__
	___X___X_____@__/__/__
	___X___X_____@__/__/__
	___X___X_____@__/__/__
5.	___X___X_____@__/__/__
	___X___X_____@__/__/__
	___X___X_____@__/__/__
	___X___X_____@__/__/__
	___X___X_____@__/__/__
6.	___X___X_____@__/__/__
	___X___X_____@__/__/__
	___X___X_____@__/__/__
	___X___X_____@__/__/__
	___X___X_____@__/__/__
7.	___X___X_____@__/__/__
	___X___X_____@__/__/__
	___X___X_____@__/__/__
	___X___X_____@__/__/__
	___X___X_____@__/__/__
8.	___X___X_____@__/__/__
	___X___X_____@__/__/__
	___X___X_____@__/__/__
	___X___X_____@__/__/__
	___X___X_____@__/__/__
9.	___X___X_____@__/__/__
	___X___X_____@__/__/__
	___X___X_____@__/__/__
	___X___X_____@__/__/__
	___X___X_____@__/__/__

CARDIO SESSION #1

TIME:_____

ACTIVITY:_____

DURATION:_____LEVEL_____

DISTANCE:_____

CALORIES BURNED:_____

ACTIVITY PULSE RATE:_____bpm

RECOVERY PULSE RATE:_____bpm

DIFFERENCE:

DAILY SLEEP TRACKER

TIME TO BED:_____

TIME UP:_____

HOURS OF SLEEP:_____

COMMENTS:_____

DAILY AB TRACKER

EXERCISE	SET X REPS X WGT
1._____	___X___X___
2._____	___X___X___
3._____	___X___X___
4._____	___X___X___
5._____	___X___X___

FITNESS CLASS

(or any physical activity-walk, jog, squash)

START:_____FINISH:_____

TYPE:_____

INSTRUCTOR:_____

ESTIMATE OF
CALORIES BURNED:

COMMENTS:_____

CARDIO SESSION #2

TIME:_____

ACTIVITY:_____

DURATION:_____LEVEL_____

DISTANCE:_____

CALORIES BURNED:_____

ACTIVITY PULSE RATE:_____bpm

RECOVERY PULSE RATE:_____bpm

DIFFERENCE:_____

COMMENTS:_____

_____

TOTAL CALORIES
BURNED TODAY:

Daily Nutrition Tracking

NUTRITION	Points Goal	CAL *option*	PROT *grams*	FAT *grams*	CARB *grams*
Meal #1 – Time: H₂O____Cups(L)					
Meal #2 – Time: H₂O____Cups(L)					
Meal #3 – Time: H₂O____Cups(L)					
Meal #4 – Time: H₂O____Cups(L)					
Meal #5 – Time: H₂O____Cups(L)					
Meal #6 – Time: H₂O____Cups(L)					

2

Food Point Total For Today:					
Difference (Goal Points Minus Actual Points)					

Daily Totals: *(Add up each nutrient column. Convert each to calories. Add all and enter in "Total Calories")*   →   g   g   g

Conversion To Calories
Multiply Total Grams of **Pro X 4** = Calories
Multiply Total Grams of **Carb X 4** = Calories
Multiply Total Grams of **Fat X 9** = Calories

Total Calories   →   cal   cal   cal

Daily Percentages: *(Divide total calories of each nutrient by the Total Number of Calories)*   →   %   %   %

Total Calories Consumed: _____
VS   **Difference**
Total Calories Burned: _____

Personal Training Log

WEIGHT TRAINING

Date:_____ Phase:_____

Start:_____ Finish:_____ Duration:_____

Day:_____ Warm Up:_____

EXERCISE	SET	X	REPS	X	WEIGHT	@	TEMPO
1.	___	X	___	X	_____	@	_/_/_
	___	X	___	X	_____	@	_/_/_
	___	X	___	X	_____	@	_/_/_
	___	X	___	X	_____	@	_/_/_
	___	X	___	X	_____	@	_/_/_
2.	___	X	___	X	_____	@	_/_/_
	___	X	___	X	_____	@	_/_/_
	___	X	___	X	_____	@	_/_/_
	___	X	___	X	_____	@	_/_/_
	___	X	___	X	_____	@	_/_/_
3.	___	X	___	X	_____	@	_/_/_
	___	X	___	X	_____	@	_/_/_
	___	X	___	X	_____	@	_/_/_
	___	X	___	X	_____	@	_/_/_
	___	X	___	X	_____	@	_/_/_
4.	___	X	___	X	_____	@	_/_/_
	___	X	___	X	_____	@	_/_/_
	___	X	___	X	_____	@	_/_/_
	___	X	___	X	_____	@	_/_/_
	___	X	___	X	_____	@	_/_/_
5.	___	X	___	X	_____	@	_/_/_
	___	X	___	X	_____	@	_/_/_
	___	X	___	X	_____	@	_/_/_
	___	X	___	X	_____	@	_/_/_
	___	X	___	X	_____	@	_/_/_
6.	___	X	___	X	_____	@	_/_/_
	___	X	___	X	_____	@	_/_/_
	___	X	___	X	_____	@	_/_/_
	___	X	___	X	_____	@	_/_/_
	___	X	___	X	_____	@	_/_/_
7.	___	X	___	X	_____	@	_/_/_
	___	X	___	X	_____	@	_/_/_
	___	X	___	X	_____	@	_/_/_
	___	X	___	X	_____	@	_/_/_
	___	X	___	X	_____	@	_/_/_
8.	___	X	___	X	_____	@	_/_/_
	___	X	___	X	_____	@	_/_/_
	___	X	___	X	_____	@	_/_/_
	___	X	___	X	_____	@	_/_/_
	___	X	___	X	_____	@	_/_/_
9.	___	X	___	X	_____	@	_/_/_
	___	X	___	X	_____	@	_/_/_
	___	X	___	X	_____	@	_/_/_
	___	X	___	X	_____	@	_/_/_
	___	X	___	X	_____	@	_/_/_

CARDIO SESSION #1

TIME:_____

ACTIVITY:_____

DURATION:_____ LEVEL_____

DISTANCE:_____

CALORIES BURNED:_____

ACTIVITY PULSE RATE:_____bpm

RECOVERY PULSE RATE:_____bpm

DIFFERENCE:

DAILY SLEEP TRACKER

TIME TO BED:_____

TIME UP:_____

HOURS OF SLEEP:_____

COMMENTS:_____

DAILY AB TRACKER

EXERCISE	SET	X	REPS	X	WGT
1._____	___	X	___	X	___
2._____	___	X	___	X	___
3._____	___	X	___	X	___
4._____	___	X	___	X	___
5._____	___	X	___	X	___

FITNESS CLASS
(or any physical activity-walk, jog, squash)

START:_____ FINISH:_____

TYPE:_____

INSTRUCTOR:_____

ESTIMATE OF
CALORIES BURNED: [   ]

COMMENTS:_____

CARDIO SESSION #2

TIME:_____

ACTIVITY:_____

DURATION:_____ LEVEL_____

DISTANCE:_____

CALORIES BURNED:_____

ACTIVITY PULSE RATE:_____bpm

RECOVERY PULSE RATE:_____bpm

DIFFERENCE:_____

COMMENTS:_____

TOTAL CALORIES
BURNED TODAY: [   ]

NUTRITION	Points Goal	CAL *option*	PROT *grams*	FAT *grams*	CARB *grams*
Meal #1 – Time: H₂O____Cups(L)					
Meal #2 – Time: H₂O____Cups(L)					
Meal #3 – Time: H₂O____Cups(L)					
Meal #4 – Time: H₂O____Cups(L)					
Meal #5 – Time: H₂O____Cups(L)					
Meal #6 – Time: H₂O____Cups(L)					

2

Food Point Total For Today:		
Difference (Goal Points Minus Actual Points)		

Daily Totals: *(Add up each nutrient column. Convert each to calories. Add all and enter in "Total Calories")*   g   g   g

Conversion To Calories	***Total***	
Multiply Total Grams of **Pro X 4** = Calories	***Calories***	
Multiply Total Grams of **Carb X 4** = Calories		
Multiply Total Grams of **Fat X 9** = Calories		cal cal cal

Daily Percentages: *(Divide total calories of each nutrient by the Total Number of Calories)*   ___%   ___%   ___%

Total Calories Consumed: _____
       VS   ***Difference***
Total Calories Burned: _____

Personal Training Log

WEIGHT TRAINING

Date:_____ Phase:_____
Start:_____ Finish:_____ Duration:_____
Day:_____ Warm Up:_____

EXERCISE	SET X REPS X WEIGHT @ TEMPO
1.	___X___X_____ @__/__/__
	___X___X_____ @__/__/__
	___X___X_____ @__/__/__
	___X___X_____ @__/__/__
	___X___X_____ @__/__/__
2.	___X___X_____ @__/__/__
	___X___X_____ @__/__/__
	___X___X_____ @__/__/__
	___X___X_____ @__/__/__
	___X___X_____ @__/__/__
3.	___X___X_____ @__/__/__
	___X___X_____ @__/__/__
	___X___X_____ @__/__/__
	___X___X_____ @__/__/__
	___X___X_____ @__/__/__
4.	___X___X_____ @__/__/__
	___X___X_____ @__/__/__
	___X___X_____ @__/__/__
	___X___X_____ @__/__/__
	___X___X_____ @__/__/__
5.	___X___X_____ @__/__/__
	___X___X_____ @__/__/__
	___X___X_____ @__/__/__
	___X___X_____ @__/__/__
	___X___X_____ @__/__/__
6.	___X___X_____ @__/__/__
	___X___X_____ @__/__/__
	___X___X_____ @__/__/__
	___X___X_____ @__/__/__
	___X___X_____ @__/__/__
7.	___X___X_____ @__/__/__
	___X___X_____ @__/__/__
	___X___X_____ @__/__/__
	___X___X_____ @__/__/__
	___X___X_____ @__/__/__
8.	___X___X_____ @__/__/__
	___X___X_____ @__/__/__
	___X___X_____ @__/__/__
	___X___X_____ @__/__/__
	___X___X_____ @__/__/__
9.	___X___X_____ @__/__/__
	___X___X_____ @__/__/__
	___X___X_____ @__/__/__
	___X___X_____ @__/__/__
	___X___X_____ @__/__/__

CARDIO SESSION #1

TIME:_____
ACTIVITY:_____
DURATION:_____ LEVEL_____
DISTANCE:_____
CALORIES BURNED:_____
ACTIVITY PULSE RATE:_____bpm
RECOVERY PULSE RATE:_____bpm
DIFFERENCE:

DAILY SLEEP TRACKER

TIME TO BED:_____
TIME UP:_____
HOURS OF SLEEP:_____
COMMENTS:_____

DAILY AB TRACKER

EXERCISE	SET X REPS X WGT
1._____	___X___X_____
2._____	___X___X_____
3._____	___X___X_____
4._____	___X___X_____
5._____	___X___X_____

FITNESS CLASS
(or any physical activity-walk, jog, squash)

START:_____ FINISH:_____
TYPE:_____
INSTRUCTOR:_____
ESTIMATE OF
CALORIES BURNED: [ ]
COMMENTS:_____

CARDIO SESSION #2

TIME:_____
ACTIVITY:_____
DURATION:_____ LEVEL_____
DISTANCE:_____
CALORIES BURNED:_____
ACTIVITY PULSE RATE:_____bpm
RECOVERY PULSE RATE:_____bpm
DIFFERENCE:_____

COMMENTS:_____
_____
TOTAL CALORIES
BURNED TODAY: [ ]

2

NUTRITION		Points Goal	CAL option	PROT grams	FAT grams	CARB grams
Meal #1 – Time:	H_2O____Cups(L)					
Meal #2 – Time:	H_2O____Cups(L)					
Meal #3 – Time:	H_2O____Cups(L)					
Meal #4 – Time:	H_2O____Cups(L)					
Meal #5 – Time:	H_2O____Cups(L)					
Meal #6 – Time:	H_2O____Cups(L)					

2

Food Point Total For Today:		
Difference (Goal Points Minus Actual Points)		

Daily Totals: (Add up each nutrient column. Convert each to calories. Add all and enter in "Total Calories")		g	g	g

Conversion To Calories Multiply Total Grams of **Pro X 4** = Calories Multiply Total Grams of **Carb X 4** = Calories Multiply Total Grams of **Fat X 9** = Calories	**Total Calories**	cal	cal	cal

Daily Percentages: (Divide total calories of each nutrient by the Total Number of Calories)	%	%	%

Total Calories Consumed:_____
            VS   **Difference**
Total Calories Burned: _____

Personal Training Log

WEIGHT TRAINING

Date:_____Phase:_____

Start:_____Finish:_____Duration:_____

Day:_____Warm Up:_____

EXERCISE	SET X REPS X WEIGHT @ TEMPO
1.	___X___X_____@__/__/__
	___X___X_____@__/__/__
	___X___X_____@__/__/__
	___X___X_____@__/__/__
	___X___X_____@__/__/__
2.	___X___X_____@__/__/__
	___X___X_____@__/__/__
	___X___X_____@__/__/
	___X___X_____@__/__/
	___X___X_____@__/__/
3.	___X___X_____@__/__/
	___X___X_____@__/__/__
	___X___X_____@__/__/__
	___X___X_____@__/__/__
	___X___X_____@__/__/
4.	___X___X_____@__/__/
	___X___X_____@__/__/
	___X___X_____@__/__/__
	___X___X_____@__/__/
	___X___X_____@__/__/
5.	___X___X_____@__/__/
	___X___X_____@__/__/
	___X___X_____@__/__/
	___X___X_____@__/__/
	___X___X_____@__/__/__
6.	___X___X_____@__/__/
	___X___X_____@__/__/
	___X___X_____@__/__/
	___X___X_____@__/__/
	___X___X_____@__/__/__
7.	___X___X_____@__/__/
	___X___X_____@__/__/
	___X___X_____@__/__/
	___X___X_____@__/__/
	___X___X_____@__/__/__
8.	___X___X_____@__/__/
	___X___X_____@__/__/
	___X___X_____@__/__/
	___X___X_____@__/__/
	___X___X_____@__/__/
9.	___X___X_____@__/__/
	___X___X_____@__/__/__
	___X___X_____@__/__/__
	___X___X_____@__/__/__
	___X___X_____@__/__/

CARDIO SESSION #1

TIME:_____

ACTIVITY:_____

DURATION:_____LEVEL_____

DISTANCE:_____

CALORIES BURNED:_____

ACTIVITY PULSE RATE:_____bpm

RECOVERY PULSE RATE:_____bpm

DIFFERENCE:

DAILY SLEEP TRACKER

TIME TO BED:_____

TIME UP:_____

HOURS OF SLEEP:_____

COMMENTS:_____

DAILY AB TRACKER

EXERCISE	SET X REPS X WGT
1._____	___X___X_____
2._____	___X___X_____
3._____	___X___X_____
4._____	___X___X_____
5._____	___X___X_____

FITNESS CLASS
(or any physical activity-walk, jog, squash)

START:_____FINISH:_____

TYPE:_____

INSTRUCTOR:_____

ESTIMATE OF
CALORIES BURNED:

COMMENTS:_____

CARDIO SESSION #2

TIME:_____

ACTIVITY:_____

DURATION:_____LEVEL_____

DISTANCE:_____

CALORIES BURNED:_____

ACTIVITY PULSE RATE:_____bpm

RECOVERY PULSE RATE:_____bpm

DIFFERENCE:

COMMENTS:_____

TOTAL CALORIES
BURNED TODAY:

NUTRITION	Points Goal	CAL *option*	PROT *grams*	FAT *grams*	CARB *grams*
Meal #1 – Time: H₂O___Cups(L)					
Meal #2 – Time: H₂O___Cups(L)					
Meal #3 – Time: H₂O___Cups(L)					
Meal #4 – Time: H₂O___Cups(L)					
Meal #5 – Time: H₂O___Cups(L)					
Meal #6 – Time: H₂O___Cups(L)					

2

Food Point Total For Today:					
Difference (Goal Points Minus Actual Points)					
Daily Totals: *(Add up each nutrient column. Convert each to calories. Add all and enter in "Total Calories")*			g	g	g
Conversion To Calories *Multiply Total Grams of **Pro X 4** = Calories* *Multiply Total Grams of **Carb X 4**=Calories* *Multiply Total Grams of **Fat X 9** = Calories*	**Total Calories**		cal	cal	cal
Daily Percentages: *(Divide total calories of each nutrient by the Total Number of Calories)*			___ %	___ %	___ %

Total Calories Consumed:_____
                    VS   **Difference**
Total Calories Burned: _____

Personal Training Log

WEIGHT TRAINING

Date:_____Phase:_____

Start:_____Finish:_____Duration:_____

Day:_____Warm Up:_____

EXERCISE	SET X REPS X WEIGHT @ TEMPO
1.	___X____X _____ @__/__/__
	___X____X _____ @__/__/__
	___X____X _____ @__/__/__
	___X____X _____ @__/__/__
	___X____X _____ @__/__/__
2.	___X____X _____ @__/__/__
	___X____X _____ @__/__/__
	___X____X _____ @__/__/__
	___X____X _____ @__/__/__
	___X____X _____ @__/__/__
3.	___X____X _____ @__/__/__
	___X____X _____ @__/__/__
	___X____X _____ @__/__/__
	___X____X _____ @__/__/__
	___X____X _____ @__/__/__
4.	___X____X _____ @__/__/__
	___X____X _____ @__/__/__
	___X____X _____ @__/__/__
	___X____X _____ @__/__/__
	___X____X _____ @__/__/__
5.	___X____X _____ @__/__/__
	___X____X _____ @__/__/__
	___X____X _____ @__/__/__
	___X____X _____ @__/__/__
	___X____X _____ @__/__/__
6.	___X____X _____ @__/__/__
	___X____X _____ @__/__/__
	___X____X _____ @__/__/__
	___X____X _____ @__/__/__
	___X____X _____ @__/__/__
7.	___X____X _____ @__/__/__
	___X____X _____ @__/__/__
	___X____X _____ @__/__/__
	___X____X _____ @__/__/__
	___X____X _____ @__/__/__
8.	___X____X _____ @__/__/__
	___X____X _____ @__/__/__
	___X____X _____ @__/__/__
	___X____X _____ @__/__/__
	___X____X _____ @__/__/__
9.	___X____X _____ @__/__/__
	___X____X _____ @__/__/__
	___X____X _____ @__/__/__
	___X____X _____ @__/__/__
	___X____X _____ @__/__/__

CARDIO SESSION #1

TIME:_____

ACTIVITY:_____

DURATION:_____LEVEL_____

DISTANCE:_____

CALORIES BURNED:_____

ACTIVITY PULSE RATE:_____bpm

RECOVERY PULSE RATE:_____bpm

DIFFERENCE:

DAILY SLEEP TRACKER

TIME TO BED:_____

TIME UP:_____

HOURS OF SLEEP:_____

COMMENTS:_____

DAILY AB TRACKER

EXERCISE	SET X REPS X WGT
1._____	___X____X_____
2._____	___X____X_____
3._____	___X____X_____
4._____	___X____X_____
5._____	___X____X_____

FITNESS CLASS
(or any physical activity-walk, jog, squash)

START:_____FINISH:_____

TYPE:_____

INSTRUCTOR:_____

ESTIMATE OF
CALORIES BURNED:

COMMENTS:_____

CARDIO SESSION #2

TIME:_____

ACTIVITY:_____

DURATION:_____LEVEL_____

DISTANCE:_____

CALORIES BURNED:_____

ACTIVITY PULSE RATE:_____bpm

RECOVERY PULSE RATE:_____bpm

DIFFERENCE:_____

COMMENTS:_____

TOTAL CALORIES
BURNED TODAY:

NUTRITION		Points Goal	CAL *option*	PROT *grams*	FAT *grams*	CARB *grams*
Meal #1 – Time:	H₂O____Cups(L)					
Meal #2 – Time:	H₂O____Cups(L)					
Meal #3 – Time:	H₂O____Cups(L)					
Meal #4 – Time:	H₂O____Cups(L)					
Meal #5 – Time:	H₂O____Cups(L)					
Meal #6 – Time:	H₂O____Cups(L)					

Food Point Total For Today:

Difference (Goal Points Minus Actual Points)

Daily Totals: (Add up each nutrient column. Convert each to calories. Add all and enter in "Total Calories")   g   g   g

Conversion To Calories
Multiply Total Grams of **Pro X 4** = Calories
Multiply Total Grams of **Carb X 4** = Calories
Multiply Total Grams of **Fat X 9** = Calories

Total Calories   cal   cal   cal

Daily Percentages: (Divide total calories of each nutrient by the Total Number of Calories)   %   %   %

Total Calories Consumed: _____
VS   **Difference**
Total Calories Burned: _____

Personal Training Log

WEIGHT TRAINING

Date:_____ Phase:_____

Start:_____ Finish:_____ Duration:_____

Day:_____ Warm Up:_____

EXERCISE	SET X REPS X WEIGHT @ TEMPO
1.	___X___X _____@__/__/__
	___X___X _____@__/__/__
	___X___X _____@__/__/__
	___X___X _____@__/__/__
	___X___X _____@__/__/__
2.	___X___X _____@__/__/__
	___X___X _____@__/__/__
	___X___X _____@__/__/__
	___X___X _____@__/__/__
	___X___X _____@__/__/__
3.	___X___X _____@__/__/__
	___X___X _____@__/__/__
	___X___X _____@__/__/__
	___X___X _____@__/__/__
	___X___X _____@__/__/__
4.	___X___X _____@__/__/__
	___X___X _____@__/__/__
	___X___X _____@__/__/__
	___X___X _____@__/__/__
	___X___X _____@__/__/__
5.	___X___X _____@__/__/__
	___X___X _____@__/__/__
	___X___X _____@__/__/__
	___X___X _____@__/__/__
	___X___X _____@__/__/__
6.	___X___X _____@__/__/__
	___X___X _____@__/__/__
	___X___X _____@__/__/__
	___X___X _____@__/__/__
	___X___X _____@__/__/__
7.	___X___X _____@__/__/__
	___X___X _____@__/__/__
	___X___X _____@__/__/__
	___X___X _____@__/__/__
	___X___X _____@__/__/__
8.	___X___X _____@__/__/__
	___X___X _____@__/__/__
	___X___X _____@__/__/__
	___X___X _____@__/__/__
	___X___X _____@__/__/__
9.	___X___X _____@__/__/__
	___X___X _____@__/__/__
	___X___X _____@__/__/__
	___X___X _____@__/__/__
	___X___X _____@__/__/__

CARDIO SESSION #1

TIME:_____

ACTIVITY:_____

DURATION:_____ LEVEL_____

DISTANCE:_____

CALORIES BURNED:_____

ACTIVITY PULSE RATE:_____bpm

RECOVERY PULSE RATE:_____bpm

DIFFERENCE:

DAILY SLEEP TRACKER

TIME TO BED:_____

TIME UP:_____

HOURS OF SLEEP:_____

COMMENTS:_____

DAILY AB TRACKER

EXERCISE	SET X REPS X WGT
1._____	___X___X_____
2._____	___X___X_____
3._____	___X___X_____
4._____	___X___X_____
5._____	___X___X_____

FITNESS CLASS
(or any physical activity-walk, jog, squash)

START:_____ FINISH:_____

TYPE:_____

INSTRUCTOR:_____

ESTIMATE OF
CALORIES BURNED:

COMMENTS:_____

CARDIO SESSION #2

TIME:_____

ACTIVITY:_____

DURATION:_____ LEVEL_____

DISTANCE:_____

CALORIES BURNED:_____

ACTIVITY PULSE RATE:_____bpm

RECOVERY PULSE RATE:_____bpm

DIFFERENCE:_____

COMMENTS:_____

TOTAL CALORIES
BURNED TODAY:

2

Daily Nutrition Tracking

NUTRITION	Points Goal	CAL *option*	PROT *grams*	FAT *grams*	CARB *grams*
Meal #1 – Time: H₂O____Cups(L)					
Meal #2 – Time: H₂O____Cups(L)					
Meal #3 – Time: H₂O____Cups(L)					
Meal #4 – Time: H₂O____Cups(L)					
Meal #5 – Time: H₂O____Cups(L)					
Meal #6 – Time: H₂O____Cups(L)					

2

Food Point Total For Today:					
Difference (Goal Points Minus Actual Points)					
Daily Totals: *(Add up each nutrient column. Convert each to calories. Add all and enter in "Total Calories")*			g	g	g

Conversion To Calories Multiply Total Grams of **Pro X 4** = Calories Multiply Total Grams of **Carb X 4**=Calories Multiply Total Grams of **Fat X 9** = Calories	**Total Calories**	cal	cal	cal

Daily Percentages: (Divide total calories of each nutrient by the Total Number of Calories)	%	%	%

Total Calories Consumed:_____

VS   *Difference*

Total Calories Burned: _____

Personal Training Log

WEIGHT TRAINING

Date:_____ Phase:_____

Start:_____ Finish:_____ Duration:_____

Day:_____ Warm Up:_____

EXERCISE	SET X REPS X WEIGHT @ TEMPO
1.	___X___X _____ @__/__/__
	___X___X _____ @__/__/__
	___X___X _____ @__/__/__
	___X___X _____ @__/__/__
	___X___X _____ @__/__/__
2.	___X___X _____ @__/__/__
	___X___X _____ @__/__/__
	___X___X _____ @__/__/__
	___X___X _____ @__/__/__
	___X___X _____ @__/__/__
3.	___X___X _____ @__/__/__
	___X___X _____ @__/__/__
	___X___X _____ @__/__/__
	___X___X _____ @__/__/__
	___X___X _____ @__/__/__
4.	___X___X _____ @__/__/__
	___X___X _____ @__/__/__
	___X___X _____ @__/__/__
	___X___X _____ @__/__/__
	___X___X _____ @__/__/__
5.	___X___X _____ @__/__/__
	___X___X _____ @__/__/__
	___X___X _____ @__/__/__
	___X___X _____ @__/__/__
	___X___X _____ @__/__/__
6.	___X___X _____ @__/__/__
	___X___X _____ @__/__/__
	___X___X _____ @__/__/__
	___X___X _____ @__/__/__
	___X___X _____ @__/__/__
7.	___X___X _____ @__/__/__
	___X___X _____ @__/__/__
	___X___X _____ @__/__/__
	___X___X _____ @__/__/__
	___X___X _____ @__/__/__
8.	___X___X _____ @__/__/__
	___X___X _____ @__/__/__
	___X___X _____ @__/__/__
	___X___X _____ @__/__/__
	___X___X _____ @__/__/__
9.	___X___X _____ @__/__/__
	___X___X _____ @__/__/__
	___X___X _____ @__/__/__
	___X___X _____ @__/__/__
	___X___X _____ @__/__/__

CARDIO SESSION #1

TIME:_____

ACTIVITY:_____

DURATION:_____LEVEL_____

DISTANCE:_____

CALORIES BURNED:_____

ACTIVITY PULSE RATE:_____bpm

RECOVERY PULSE RATE:_____bpm

DIFFERENCE:

DAILY SLEEP TRACKER

TIME TO BED:_____

TIME UP:_____

HOURS OF SLEEP:_____

COMMENTS:_____

DAILY AB TRACKER

EXERCISE	SET X REPS X WGT
1._____	___X___X____
2._____	___X___X____
3._____	___X___X____
4._____	___X___X____
5._____	___X___X____

FITNESS CLASS
(or any physical activity-walk, jog, squash)

START:_____FINISH:_____

TYPE:_____

INSTRUCTOR:_____

ESTIMATE OF
CALORIES BURNED:

COMMENTS:_____

CARDIO SESSION #2

TIME:_____

ACTIVITY:_____

DURATION:_____LEVEL_____

DISTANCE:_____

CALORIES BURNED:_____

ACTIVITY PULSE RATE:_____bpm

RECOVERY PULSE RATE:_____bpm

DIFFERENCE:_____

COMMENTS:_____

TOTAL CALORIES
BURNED TODAY:

NUTRITION	Points Goal	CAL option	PROT grams	FAT grams	CARB grams
Meal #1 – Time: H₂O___Cups(L)					
Meal #2 – Time: H₂O___Cups(L)					
Meal #3 – Time: H₂O___Cups(L)					
Meal #4 – Time: H₂O___Cups(L)					
Meal #5 – Time: H₂O___Cups(L)					
Meal #6 – Time: H₂O___Cups(L)					

Food Point Total For Today:

Difference (Goal Points Minus Actual Points)

Daily Totals: (Add up each nutrient column. Convert each to calories. Add all and enter in "Total Calories")   g   g   g

Conversion To Calories
Multiply Total Grams of **Pro X 4** = Calories
Multiply Total Grams of **Carb X 4** = Calories
Multiply Total Grams of **Fat X 9** = Calories

Total Calories   cal   cal   cal

Daily Percentages: (Divide total calories of each nutrient by the Total Number of Calories)   %   %   %

Total Calories Consumed: ___
     VS   **Difference**
Total Calories Burned: ___

2

Personal Training Log

WEIGHT TRAINING

Date:_____ Phase:_____

Start:_____ Finish:_____ Duration:_____

Day:_____ Warm Up:_____

EXERCISE	SET X REPS X WEIGHT @ TEMPO
1.	___X___X_____@__/__/__ ___X___X_____@__/__/__ ___X___X_____@__/__/__ ___X___X_____@__/__/__ ___X___X_____@__/__/__
2.	___X___X_____@__/__/__ ___X___X_____@__/__/__ ___X___X_____@__/__/__ ___X___X_____@__/__/__ ___X___X_____@__/__/__
3.	___X___X_____@__/__/__ ___X___X_____@__/__/__ ___X___X_____@__/__/__ ___X___X_____@__/__/__ ___X___X_____@__/__/__
4.	___X___X_____@__/__/__ ___X___X_____@__/__/__ ___X___X_____@__/__/__ ___X___X_____@__/__/__ ___X___X_____@__/__/__
5.	___X___X_____@__/__/__ ___X___X_____@__/__/__ ___X___X_____@__/__/__ ___X___X_____@__/__/__ ___X___X_____@__/__/__
6.	___X___X_____@__/__/__ ___X___X_____@__/__/__ ___X___X_____@__/__/__ ___X___X_____@__/__/__ ___X___X_____@__/__/__
7.	___X___X_____@__/__/__ ___X___X_____@__/__/__ ___X___X_____@__/__/__ ___X___X_____@__/__/__ ___X___X_____@__/__/__
8.	___X___X_____@__/__/__ ___X___X_____@__/__/__ ___X___X_____@__/__/__ ___X___X_____@__/__/__ ___X___X_____@__/__/__
9.	___X___X_____@__/__/__ ___X___X_____@__/__/__ ___X___X_____@__/__/__ ___X___X_____@__/__/__ ___X___X_____@__/__/__

2

CARDIO SESSION #1

TIME:_____

ACTIVITY:_____

DURATION:_____ LEVEL_____

DISTANCE:_____

CALORIES BURNED:_____

ACTIVITY PULSE RATE:_____ bpm

RECOVERY PULSE RATE:_____ bpm

DIFFERENCE:

DAILY SLEEP TRACKER

TIME TO BED:_____

TIME UP:_____

HOURS OF SLEEP:_____

COMMENTS:_____

DAILY AB TRACKER

EXERCISE	SET X REPS X WGT
1._____	___X___X_____
2._____	___X___X_____
3._____	___X___X_____
4._____	___X___X_____
5._____	___X___X_____

FITNESS CLASS
(or any physical activity-walk, jog, squash)

START:_____ FINISH:_____

TYPE:_____

INSTRUCTOR:_____

ESTIMATE OF
CALORIES BURNED: [____]

COMMENTS:_____

CARDIO SESSION #2

TIME:_____

ACTIVITY:_____

DURATION:_____ LEVEL_____

DISTANCE:_____

CALORIES BURNED:_____

ACTIVITY PULSE RATE:_____ bpm

RECOVERY PULSE RATE:_____ bpm

DIFFERENCE:_____

COMMENTS:_____

TOTAL CALORIES
BURNED TODAY: [____]

Daily Nutrition Tracking

NUTRITION	Points Goal	CAL *option*	PROT *grams*	FAT *grams*	CARB *grams*
Meal #1 – Time: H₂O_____Cups(L)					
Meal #2 – Time: H₂O_____Cups(L)					
Meal #3 – Time: H₂O_____Cups(L)					
Meal #4 – Time: H₂O_____Cups(L)					
Meal #5 – Time: H₂O_____Cups(L)					
Meal #6 – Time: H₂O_____Cups(L)					

2

Food Point Total For Today:				
Difference (Goal Points Minus Actual Points)				
Daily Totals:(Add up each nutrient column. Convert each to calories. Add all and enter in "Total Calories")		**g**	**g**	**g**

Conversion To Calories Multiply Total Grams of **Pro X 4** = Calories Multiply Total Grams of **Carb X 4**=Calories Multiply Total Grams of **Fat X 9** = Calories	**Total Calories**	**cal**	**cal**	**cal**

Daily Percentages: (Divide total calories of each nutrient by the Total Number of Calories)		___ **%**	___ **%**	___ **%**

Total Calories Consumed:_____

         VS   **Difference**

Total Calories Burned: _____

Personal Training Log

WEIGHT TRAINING

Date:_____ Phase:_____

Start:_____ Finish:_____ Duration:_____

Day:_____ Warm Up:_____

EXERCISE	SET X REPS X WEIGHT @ TEMPO
1.	___X___X_____@__/__/__
	___X___X_____@__/__/__
	___X___X_____@__/__/__
	___X___X_____@__/__/__
	___X___X_____@__/__/__
2.	___X___X_____@__/__/__
	___X___X_____@__/__/__
	___X___X_____@__/__/__
	___X___X_____@__/__/__
	___X___X_____@__/__/__
3.	___X___X_____@__/__/__
	___X___X_____@__/__/__
	___X___X_____@__/__/__
	___X___X_____@__/__/__
	___X___X_____@__/__/__
4.	___X___X_____@__/__/__
	___X___X_____@__/__/__
	___X___X_____@__/__/__
	___X___X_____@__/__/__
	___X___X_____@__/__/__
5.	___X___X_____@__/__/__
	___X___X_____@__/__/__
	___X___X_____@__/__/__
	___X___X_____@__/__/__
	___X___X_____@__/__/__
6.	___X___X_____@__/__/__
	___X___X_____@__/__/__
	___X___X_____@__/__/__
	___X___X_____@__/__/__
	___X___X_____@__/__/__
7.	___X___X_____@__/__/__
	___X___X_____@__/__/__
	___X___X_____@__/__/__
	___X___X_____@__/__/__
	___X___X_____@__/__/__
8.	___X___X_____@__/__/__
	___X___X_____@__/__/__
	___X___X_____@__/__/__
	___X___X_____@__/__/__
	___X___X_____@__/__/__
9.	___X___X_____@__/__/__
	___X___X_____@__/__/__
	___X___X_____@__/__/__
	___X___X_____@__/__/__
	___X___X_____@__/__/__

CARDIO SESSION #1

TIME:_____

ACTIVITY:_____

DURATION:_____LEVEL_____

DISTANCE:_____

CALORIES BURNED:_____

ACTIVITY PULSE RATE:_____bpm

RECOVERY PULSE RATE:_____bpm

DIFFERENCE:

DAILY SLEEP TRACKER

TIME TO BED:_____

TIME UP:_____

HOURS OF SLEEP:_____

COMMENTS:_____

DAILY AB TRACKER

EXERCISE	SET X REPS X WGT
1._____	___X___X_____
2._____	___X___X_____
3._____	___X___X_____
4._____	___X___X_____
5._____	___X___X_____

FITNESS CLASS
(or any physical activity-walk, jog, squash)

START:_____FINISH:_____

TYPE:_____

INSTRUCTOR:_____

ESTIMATE OF
CALORIES BURNED:

COMMENTS:_____

CARDIO SESSION #2

TIME:_____

ACTIVITY:_____

DURATION:_____LEVEL_____

DISTANCE:_____

CALORIES BURNED:_____

ACTIVITY PULSE RATE:_____bpm

RECOVERY PULSE RATE:_____bpm

DIFFERENCE: _____

COMMENTS:_____

TOTAL CALORIES
BURNED TODAY:

2

Daily Nutrition Tracking

NUTRITION	Points Goal	CAL *option*	PROT *grams*	FAT *grams*	CARB *grams*
Meal #1 – Time: H₂O____Cups(L)					
Meal #2 – Time: H₂O____Cups(L)					
Meal #3 – Time: H₂O____Cups(L)					
Meal #4 – Time: H₂O____Cups(L)					
Meal #5 – Time: H₂O____Cups(L)					
Meal #6 Time: H₂O____Cups(L)					

2

Food Point Total For Today:		
Difference (Goal Points Minus Actual Points)		

Daily Totals: *(Add up each nutrient column. Convert each to calories. Add all and enter in "Total Calories")*   g   g   g

Conversion To Calories
Multiply Total Grams of **Pro X 4** = Calories
Multiply Total Grams of **Carb X 4**=Calories
Multiply Total Grams of **Fat X 9** = Calories

Total Calories   cal   cal   cal

Daily Percentages: (Divide total calories of each nutrient by the Total Number of Calories)   ___%   ___%   ___%

Total Calories Consumed:_____
VS   **Difference**
Total Calories Burned: _____

Personal Training Log

WEIGHT TRAINING

Date:_____ Phase:_____

Start:_____ Finish:_____ Duration:_____

Day:_____ Warm Up:_____

EXERCISE	SET X REPS X WEIGHT @ TEMPO
1.	___X___X ___ @__/__/__
	___X___X ___ @__/__/__
	___X___X ___ @__/__/__
	___X___X ___ @__/__/__
	___X___X ___ @__/__/__
2.	___X___X ___ @__/__/__
	___X___X ___ @__/__/__
	___X___X ___ @__/__/__
	___X___X ___ @__/__/__
	___X___X ___ @__/__/__
3.	___X___X ___ @__/__/__
	___X___X ___ @__/__/__
	___X___X ___ @__/__/__
	___X___X ___ @__/__/__
	___X___X ___ @__/__/__
4.	___X___X ___ @__/__/__
	___X___X ___ @__/__/__
	___X___X ___ @__/__/__
	___X___X ___ @__/__/__
	___X___X ___ @__/__/__
5.	___X___X ___ @__/__/__
	___X___X ___ @__/__/__
	___X___X ___ @__/__/__
	___X___X ___ @__/__/__
	___X___X ___ @__/__/__
6.	___X___X ___ @__/__/__
	___X___X ___ @__/__/__
	___X___X ___ @__/__/__
	___X___X ___ @__/__/__
	___X___X ___ @__/__/__
7.	___X___X ___ @__/__/__
	___X___X ___ @__/__/__
	___X___X ___ @__/__/__
	___X___X ___ @__/__/__
	___X___X ___ @__/__/__
8.	___X___X ___ @__/__/__
	___X___X ___ @__/__/__
	___X___X ___ @__/__/__
	___X___X ___ @__/__/__
	___X___X ___ @__/__/__
9.	___X___X ___ @__/__/__
	___X___X ___ @__/__/__
	___X___X ___ @__/__/__
	___X___X ___ @__/__/__
	___X___X ___ @__/__/__

CARDIO SESSION #1

TIME:_____

ACTIVITY:_____

DURATION:_____ LEVEL_____

DISTANCE:_____

CALORIES BURNED:_____

ACTIVITY PULSE RATE:_____bpm

RECOVERY PULSE RATE:_____bpm

DIFFERENCE:

DAILY SLEEP TRACKER

TIME TO BED:_____

TIME UP:_____

HOURS OF SLEEP:_____

COMMENTS:_____

DAILY AB TRACKER

EXERCISE	SET X REPS X WGT
1._____	___X___X___
2._____	___X___X___
3._____	___X___X___
4._____	___X___X___
5._____	___X___X___

FITNESS CLASS

(or any physical activity-walk, jog, squash)

START:_____ FINISH:_____

TYPE:_____

INSTRUCTOR:_____

ESTIMATE OF
CALORIES BURNED: [ ]

COMMENTS:_____

CARDIO SESSION #2

TIME:_____

ACTIVITY:_____

DURATION:_____ LEVEL_____

DISTANCE:_____

CALORIES BURNED:_____

ACTIVITY PULSE RATE:_____bpm

RECOVERY PULSE RATE:_____bpm

DIFFERENCE:_____

COMMENTS:_____
_____

TOTAL CALORIES
BURNED TODAY: [ ]

NUTRITION	Points Goal	CAL *option*	PROT *grams*	FAT *grams*	CARB *grams*
Meal #1 – Time: H₂O____Cups(L)					
Meal #2 – Time: H₂O____Cups(L)					
Meal #3 – Time: H₂O____Cups(L)					
Meal #4 – Time: H₂O____Cups(L)					
Meal #5 – Time: H₂O____Cups(L)					
Meal #6 – Time: H₂O____Cups(L)					
Food Point Total For Today:					
Difference (Goal Points Minus Actual Points)					
Daily Totals: (Add up each nutrient column. Convert each to calories. Add all and enter in "Total Calories")			g	g	g
Conversion To Calories Multiply Total Grams of **Pro X 4** = Calories / Multiply Total Grams of **Carb X 4**=Calories / Multiply Total Grams of **Fat X 9** = Calories	**Total Calories**		cal	cal	cal
Daily Percentages: (Divide total calories of each nutrient by the Total Number of Calories)			___ %	___ %	___ %

Total Calories Consumed:_____

                 VS   **Difference**

Total Calories Burned: _____

Personal Training Log

WEIGHT TRAINING

Date:_____ Phase:_____

Start:_____ Finish:_____ Duration:_____

Day:_____ Warm Up:_____

EXERCISE	SET X REPS X WEIGHT @ TEMPO
1.	___X___X____@__/__/__
	___X___X____@__/__/__
	___X___X____@__/__/__
	___X___X____@__/__/__
	___X___X____@__/__/__
2.	___X___X____@__/__/__
	___X___X____@__/__/__
	___X___X____@__/__/__
	___X___X____@__/__/__
	___X___X____@__/__/__
3.	___X___X____@__/__/__
	___X___X____@__/__/__
	___X___X____@__/__/__
	___X___X____@__/__/__
	___X___X____@__/__/__
4.	___X___X____@__/__/__
	___X___X____@__/__/__
	___X___X____@__/__/__
	___X___X____@__/__/__
	___X___X____@__/__/__
5.	___X___X____@__/__/__
	___X___X____@__/__/__
	___X___X____@__/__/__
	___X___X____@__/__/__
	___X___X____@__/__/__
6.	___X___X____@__/__/__
	___X___X____@__/__/__
	___X___X____@__/__/__
	___X___X____@__/__/__
	___X___X____@__/__/__
7.	___X___X____@__/__/__
	___X___X____@__/__/__
	___X___X____@__/__/__
	___X___X____@__/__/__
	___X___X____@__/__/__
8.	___X___X____@__/__/__
	___X___X____@__/__/__
	___X___X____@__/__/__
	___X___X____@__/__/__
	___X___X____@__/__/__
9.	___X___X____@__/__/__
	___X___X____@__/__/__
	___X___X____@__/__/__
	___X___X____@__/__/__
	___X___X____@__/__/__

2

CARDIO SESSION #1

TIME:_____

ACTIVITY:_____

DURATION:_____ LEVEL_____

DISTANCE:_____

CALORIES BURNED:_____

ACTIVITY PULSE RATE:_____bpm

RECOVERY PULSE RATE:_____bpm

DIFFERENCE:

DAILY SLEEP TRACKER

TIME TO BED:_____

TIME UP:_____

HOURS OF SLEEP:_____

COMMENTS:_____

DAILY AB TRACKER

EXERCISE	SET X	REPS X	WGT
1._____	___X	___X	____
2._____	___X	___X	____
3._____	___X	___X	____
4._____	___X	___X	____
5._____	___X	___X	____

FITNESS CLASS

(or any physical activity-walk, jog, squash)

START:_____ FINISH:_____

TYPE:_____

INSTRUCTOR:_____

ESTIMATE OF
CALORIES BURNED:

COMMENTS:_____

CARDIO SESSION #2

TIME:_____

ACTIVITY:_____

DURATION:_____ LEVEL_____

DISTANCE:_____

CALORIES BURNED:_____

ACTIVITY PULSE RATE:_____bpm

RECOVERY PULSE RATE:_____bpm

DIFFERENCE:_____

COMMENTS:_____

TOTAL CALORIES
BURNED TODAY:

Daily Nutrition Tracking

NUTRITION	Points Goal	CAL *option*	PROT *grams*	FAT *grams*	CARB *grams*
Meal #1 – Time: H₂O____Cups(L)					
Meal #2 – Time: H₂O____Cups(L)					
Meal #3 – Time: H₂O____Cups(L)					
Meal #4 – Time: H₂O____Cups(L)					
Meal #5 – Time: H₂O____Cups(L)					
Meal #6 – Time: H₂O____Cups(L)					

2

Food Point Total For Today:		
Difference (Goal Points Minus Actual Points)		

Daily Totals: *(Add up each nutrient column. Convert each to calories. Add all and enter in "Total Calories")* — g | g | g

Conversion To Calories
Multiply Total Grams of **Pro X 4** = Calories
Multiply Total Grams of **Carb X 4**=Calories
Multiply Total Grams of **Fat X 9** = Calories

Total Calories — cal | cal | cal

Daily Percentages: (Divide total calories of each nutrient by the Total Number of Calories) — % | % | %

Total Calories Consumed:_____
VS   **Difference**
Total Calories Burned: _____

Personal Training Log

WEIGHT TRAINING

Date:_____ Phase:_____

Start:_____ Finish:_____ Duration:_____

Day:_____ Warm Up:_____

EXERCISE	SET X REPS X WEIGHT @ TEMPO
1.	___X___X_____@___/___/___
	___X___X_____@___/___/___
	___X___X_____@___/___/___
	___X___X_____@___/___/___
	___X___X_____@___/___/___
2.	___X___X_____@___/___/___
	___X___X_____@___/___/___
	___X___X_____@___/___/___
	___X___X_____@___/___/___
	___X___X_____@___/___/___
3.	___X___X_____@___/___/___
	___X___X_____@___/___/___
	___X___X_____@___/___/___
	___X___X_____@___/___/___
	___X___X_____@___/___/___
4.	___X___X_____@___/___/___
	___X___X_____@___/___/___
	___X___X_____@___/___/___
	___X___X_____@___/___/___
	___X___X_____@___/___/___
5.	___X___X_____@___/___/___
	___X___X_____@___/___/___
	___X___X_____@___/___/___
	___X___X_____@___/___/___
	___X___X_____@___/___/___
6.	___X___X_____@___/___/___
	___X___X_____@___/___/___
	___X___X_____@___/___/___
	___X___X_____@___/___/___
	___X___X_____@___/___/___
7.	___X___X_____@___/___/___
	___X___X_____@___/___/___
	___X___X_____@___/___/___
	___X___X_____@___/___/___
	___X___X_____@___/___/___
8.	___X___X_____@___/___/___
	___X___X_____@___/___/___
	___X___X_____@___/___/___
	___X___X_____@___/___/___
	___X___X_____@___/___/___
9.	___X___X_____@___/___/___
	___X___X_____@___/___/___
	___X___X_____@___/___/___
	___X___X_____@___/___/___
	___X___X_____@___/___/___

CARDIO SESSION #1

TIME:_____

ACTIVITY:_____

DURATION:_____LEVEL_____

DISTANCE:_____

CALORIES BURNED:_____

ACTIVITY PULSE RATE:_____bpm

RECOVERY PULSE RATE:_____bpm

DIFFERENCE:

DAILY SLEEP TRACKER

TIME TO BED:_____

TIME UP:_____

HOURS OF SLEEP:_____

COMMENTS:_____

DAILY AB TRACKER

EXERCISE	SET X REPS X WGT
1._____	___X___X_____
2._____	___X___X_____
3._____	___X___X_____
4._____	___X___X_____
5._____	___X___X_____

FITNESS CLASS
(or any physical activity-walk, jog, squash)

START:_____FINISH:_____

TYPE:_____

INSTRUCTOR:_____

ESTIMATE OF
CALORIES BURNED:

COMMENTS:_____

CARDIO SESSION #2

TIME:_____

ACTIVITY:_____

DURATION:_____LEVEL_____

DISTANCE:_____

CALORIES BURNED:_____

ACTIVITY PULSE RATE:_____bpm

RECOVERY PULSE RATE:_____bpm

DIFFERENCE:_____

COMMENTS:_____

_____

TOTAL CALORIES
BURNED TODAY:

NUTRITION	Points Goal	CAL option	PROT grams	FAT grams	CARB grams
Meal #1 – Time: H_2O____Cups(L)					
Meal #2 – Time: H_2O____Cups(L)					
Meal #3 – Time: H_2O____Cups(L)					
Meal #4 – Time: H_2O____Cups(L)					
Meal #5 – Time: H_2O____Cups(L)					
Meal #6 – Time: H_2O____Cups(L)					

2

Food Point Total For Today:			
Difference (Goal Points Minus Actual Points)			

	PROT	FAT	CARB
Daily Totals: *(Add up each nutrient column. Convert each to calories. Add all and enter in "Total Calories")*	g	g	g

Conversion To Calories	***Total Calories***			
Multiply Total Grams of **Pro X 4** *= Calories* *Multiply Total Grams of* **Carb X 4**=*Calories* *Multiply Total Grams of* **Fat X 9** *= Calories*		cal	cal	cal

Daily Percentages: *(Divide total calories of each nutrient by the Total Number of Calories)*	%	%	%

Total Calories Consumed:_____

VS   ***Difference***

Total Calories Burned: _____

Personal Training Log

WEIGHT TRAINING

Date:_____ Phase:_____

Start:_____ Finish:_____ Duration:_____

Day:_____ Warm Up:_____

EXERCISE	SET X REPS X WEIGHT @ TEMPO
1.	___X___X_____@__/__/__
	___X___X_____@__/__/__
	___X___X_____@__/__/__
	___X___X_____@__/__/__
	___X___X_____@__/__/__
2.	___X___X_____@__/__/__
	___X___X_____@__/__/__
	___X___X_____@__/__/__
	___X___X_____@__/__/__
	___X___X_____@__/__/__
3.	___X___X_____@__/__/__
	___X___X_____@__/__/__
	___X___X_____@__/__/__
	___X___X_____@__/__/__
	___X___X_____@__/__/__
4.	___X___X_____@__/__/__
	___X___X_____@__/__/__
	___X___X_____@__/__/__
	___X___X_____@__/__/__
	___X___X_____@__/__/__
5.	___X___X_____@__/__/__
	___X___X_____@__/__/__
	___X___X_____@__/__/__
	___X___X_____@__/__/__
	___X___X_____@__/__/__
6.	___X___X_____@__/__/__
	___X___X_____@__/__/__
	___X___X_____@__/__/__
	___X___X_____@__/__/__
	___X___X_____@__/__/__
7.	___X___X_____@__/__/__
	___X___X_____@__/__/__
	___X___X_____@__/__/__
	___X___X_____@__/__/__
	___X___X_____@__/__/__
8.	___X___X_____@__/__/__
	___X___X_____@__/__/__
	___X___X_____@__/__/__
	___X___X_____@__/__/__
	___X___X_____@__/__/__
9.	___X___X_____@__/__/__
	___X___X_____@__/__/__
	___X___X_____@__/__/__
	___X___X_____@__/__/__
	___X___X_____@__/__/__

CARDIO SESSION #1

TIME:_____

ACTIVITY:_____

DURATION:_____ LEVEL_____

DISTANCE:_____

CALORIES BURNED:_____

ACTIVITY PULSE RATE:_____ bpm

RECOVERY PULSE RATE:_____ bpm

DIFFERENCE:

DAILY SLEEP TRACKER

TIME TO BED:_____

TIME UP:_____

HOURS OF SLEEP:_____

COMMENTS:_____

DAILY AB TRACKER

EXERCISE	SET X REPS X WGT
1._____	___X___X_____
2._____	___X___X_____
3._____	___X___X_____
4._____	___X___X_____
5._____	___X___X_____

FITNESS CLASS
(or any physical activity-walk, jog, squash)

START:_____ FINISH:_____

TYPE:_____

INSTRUCTOR:_____

ESTIMATE OF
CALORIES BURNED: [   ]

COMMENTS:_____

CARDIO SESSION #2

TIME:_____

ACTIVITY:_____

DURATION:_____ LEVEL_____

DISTANCE:_____

CALORIES BURNED:_____

ACTIVITY PULSE RATE:_____ bpm

RECOVERY PULSE RATE:_____ bpm

DIFFERENCE:_____

COMMENTS:_____

TOTAL CALORIES
BURNED TODAY: [   ]

Daily Nutrition Tracking

NUTRITION	Points Goal	CAL *option*	PROT *grams*	FAT *grams*	CARB *grams*
Meal #1 – Time:　　H₂O___Cups(L)					
Meal #2 – Time:　　H₂O___Cups(L)					
Meal #3 – Time:　　H₂O___Cups(L)					
Meal #4 – Time:　　H₂O___Cups(L)					
Meal #5 – Time:　　H₂O___Cups(L)					
Meal #6 – Time:　　H₂O___Cups(L)					
Food Point Total For Today:					
Difference *(Goal Points Minus Actual Points)*					
Daily Totals: *(Add up each nutrient column. Convert each to calories. Add all and enter in "Total Calories")*			g	g	g
Conversion To Calories *Multiply Total Grams of **Pro X 4** = Calories* *Multiply Total Grams of **Carb X 4**=Calories* *Multiply Total Grams of **Fat X 9** = Calories*	***Total Calories***		cal	cal	cal
Daily Percentages: *(Divide total calories of each nutrient by the Total Number of Calories)*			__ %	__ %	__ %

2

Total Calories Consumed:___

　　　　　VS　　　　　　　　***Difference***

Total Calories Burned:　___

Progress Evaluation

Did you meet your goals for this cycle?　　　　　Yes ☐　　No ☐

If not, what prevented you from reaching your goals?

_____

_____

_____

_____

State the positive changes that occurred during this cycle even if you didn't meet all your goals:

_____

_____

_____

_____

What do you plan to do differently during the next cycle?

_____

_____

_____

Personal Trainers/Teachers Evaluation

_____

_____

_____

_____

_____

_____

Enter Cycle

3

Personal Fitness Evaluation

Date:_____Height:_____Weight:_____Age:_____

Medical History:_____

_____

TESTING:

Resting Heart Rate:_____bpm   Blood Pressure:_____/_____   Body Fat:_____%

Flexibility:_____   Push Ups:_____   Sit Ups:_____   Chin Ups:_____

Other Required Tests & Results:

1._____ [ ]   2._____ [ ]   3._____ [ ]

4._____ [ ]   5._____ [ ]   6._____ [ ]

WAIST TO HIP RATIO:

Waist:_____ Divided by Hips:_____ = [ ]   Women: 0.8 or less
Men: 0.95 or less

GOALS FOR THIS CYCLE:

1._____   3._____

2._____   4._____

YOUR PLAN TO ACHIEVE YOUR GOALS:
Be very specific in your plan, for example you may want to increase your cardio sessions from 20 to 25 minutes or you may want to increase your daily water intake by 1 glass. State this in your plan. Be careful to make your goals REALISTIC and ATTAINABLE. Keep in mind you do not have to use all five spaces provided. Keep it simple!

1._____

2._____

3._____

4._____

5._____

3

Weight Training Program:

Day 1	Tempo		Day 2	Tempo
1._____	_/_/_	1._____		_/_/_
2._____	_/_/_	2._____		_/_/_
3._____	_/_/_	3._____		_/_/_
4._____	_/_/_	4._____		_/_/_
5._____	_/_/_	5._____		_/_/_
6._____	_/_/_	6._____		_/_/_
7._____	_/_/_	7._____		_/_/_
8._____	_/_/_	8._____		_/_/_
9._____	_/_/_	9._____		_/_/_

Aerobic Exercise Plan:

Type:_____ ___to___ x per week @____ to____min/session

Suggested Training Heart Rate: _____ to_____ beats/min

Aerobic Class Recommendation: _____

Current Eating Habits
(Typical Day)

Breakfast:_____

Snack:_____

Lunch: _____

Snack:_____

Dinner:_____

Evening Snack: _____

Suggested Changes to Eating Habits

Meal 1:_____

Meal 2: _____

Meal 3: _____

Meal 4: _____

Meal 5: _____

Meal 6: _____

3

Photograph - Start

Date Photograph taken: _____

Weight: _____ % Body Fat: _____

PLACE PHOTO
HERE

3

Photograph - End of Cycle #3

Date Photograph taken: _____

Weight: _____ % Body Fat: _____

PLACE PHOTO
HERE

3

Personal Training Log

WEIGHT TRAINING

Date:_____ Phase:_____

Start:_____ Finish:_____ Duration:_____

Day:_____ Warm Up:_____

EXERCISE	SET X REPS X WEIGHT @ TEMPO
1.	___ X ___ X ___ @ _/_/_
	___ X ___ X ___ @ _/_/_
	___ X ___ X ___ @ _/_/_
	___ X ___ X ___ @ _/_/_
	___ X ___ X ___ @ _/_/_
2.	___ X ___ X ___ @ _/_/_
	___ X ___ X ___ @ _/_/_
	___ X ___ X ___ @ _/_/_
	___ X ___ X ___ @ _/_/_
	___ X ___ X ___ @ _/_/_
3.	___ X ___ X ___ @ _/_/_
	___ X ___ X ___ @ _/_/_
	___ X ___ X ___ @ _/_/_
	___ X ___ X ___ @ _/_/_
	___ X ___ X ___ @ _/_/_
4.	___ X ___ X ___ @ _/_/_
	___ X ___ X ___ @ _/_/_
	___ X ___ X ___ @ _/_/_
	___ X ___ X ___ @ _/_/_
	___ X ___ X ___ @ _/_/_
5.	___ X ___ X ___ @ _/_/_
	___ X ___ X ___ @ _/_/_
	___ X ___ X ___ @ _/_/_
	___ X ___ X ___ @ _/_/_
	___ X ___ X ___ @ _/_/_
6.	___ X ___ X ___ @ _/_/_
	___ X ___ X ___ @ _/_/_
	___ X ___ X ___ @ _/_/_
	___ X ___ X ___ @ _/_/_
	___ X ___ X ___ @ _/_/_
7.	___ X ___ X ___ @ _/_/_
	___ X ___ X ___ @ _/_/_
	___ X ___ X ___ @ _/_/_
	___ X ___ X ___ @ _/_/_
	___ X ___ X ___ @ _/_/_
8.	___ X ___ X ___ @ _/_/_
	___ X ___ X ___ @ _/_/_
	___ X ___ X ___ @ _/_/_
	___ X ___ X ___ @ _/_/_
	___ X ___ X ___ @ _/_/_
9.	___ X ___ X ___ @ _/_/_
	___ X ___ X ___ @ _/_/_
	___ X ___ X ___ @ _/_/_
	___ X ___ X ___ @ _/_/_
	___ X ___ X ___ @ _/_/_

3

CARDIO SESSION #1

TIME:_____

ACTIVITY:_____

DURATION:_____ LEVEL_____

DISTANCE:_____

CALORIES BURNED:_____

ACTIVITY PULSE RATE:_____ bpm

RECOVERY PULSE RATE:_____ bpm

DIFFERENCE:

DAILY SLEEP TRACKER

TIME TO BED:_____

TIME UP:_____

HOURS OF SLEEP:_____

COMMENTS:_____

DAILY AB TRACKER

EXERCISE	SET X REPS X WGT
1._____	___ X ___ X ___
2._____	___ X ___ X ___
3._____	___ X ___ X ___
4._____	___ X ___ X ___
5._____	___ X ___ X ___

FITNESS CLASS
(or any physical activity-walk, jog, squash)

START:_____ FINISH:_____

TYPE:_____

INSTRUCTOR:_____

ESTIMATE OF
CALORIES BURNED: [____]

COMMENTS:_____

CARDIO SESSION #2

TIME:_____

ACTIVITY:_____

DURATION:_____ LEVEL_____

DISTANCE:_____

CALORIES BURNED:_____

ACTIVITY PULSE RATE:_____ bpm

RECOVERY PULSE RATE:_____ bpm

DIFFERENCE:_____

COMMENTS:_____

_____

TOTAL CALORIES
BURNED TODAY: [____]

NUTRITION	Points Goal	CAL *option*	PROT *grams*	FAT *grams*	CARB *grams*
Meal #1 – Time: H₂O_____Cups(L)					
Meal #2 – Time: H₂O_____Cups(L)					
Meal #3 – Time: H₂O_____Cups(L)					
Meal #4 – Time: H₂O_____Cups(L)					
Meal #5 – Time: H₂O_____Cups(L)					
Meal #6 – Time: H₂O_____Cups(L)					

Food Point Total For Today:		
Difference (Goal Points Minus Actual Points)		

3

Daily Totals: *(Add up each nutrient column. Convert each to calories. Add all and enter in "Total Calories")*		g	g	g
Conversion To Calories Multiply Total Grams of **Pro X 4** = Calories Multiply Total Grams of **Carb X 4**=Calories Multiply Total Grams of **Fat X 9** = Calories	**Total Calories**	cal	cal	cal
Daily Percentages: (Divide total calories of each nutrient by the Total Number of Calories)		___ %	___ %	___ %

Total Calories Consumed:_____
              VS   **Difference**
Total Calories Burned: _____

Personal Training Log

WEIGHT TRAINING

Date:_____Phase:_____

Start:_____Finish:_____Duration:_____

Day:_____Warm Up:_____

EXERCISE	SET X REPS X WEIGHT @ TEMPO
1.	___X_____X_____@__/__/__
	___X_____X_____@__/__/__
	___X_____X_____@__/__/__
	___X_____X_____@__/__/__
	___X_____X_____@__/__/__
2.	___X_____X_____@__/__/__
	___X_____X_____@__/__/__
	___X_____X_____@__/__/__
	___X_____X_____@__/__/__
	___X_____X_____@__/__/__
3.	___X_____X_____@__/__/__
	___X_____X_____@__/__/__
	___X_____X_____@__/__/__
	___X_____X_____@__/__/__
	___X_____X_____@__/__/__
4.	___X_____X_____@__/__/__
	___X_____X_____@__/__/__
	___X_____X_____@__/__/__
	___X_____X_____@__/__/__
	___X_____X_____@__/__/__
5.	___X_____X_____@__/__/__
	___X_____X_____@__/__/__
	___X_____X_____@__/__/__
	___X_____X_____@__/__/__
	___X_____X_____@__/__/__
6.	___X_____X_____@__/__/__
	___X_____X_____@__/__/__
	___X_____X_____@__/__/__
	___X_____X_____@__/__/__
	___X_____X_____@__/__/__
7.	___X_____X_____@__/__/__
	___X_____X_____@__/__/__
	___X_____X_____@__/__/__
	___X_____X_____@__/__/__
	___X_____X_____@__/__/__
8.	___X_____X_____@__/__/__
	___X_____X_____@__/__/__
	___X_____X_____@__/__/__
	___X_____X_____@__/__/__
	___X_____X_____@__/__/__
9.	___X_____X_____@__/__/__
	___X_____X_____@__/__/__
	___X_____X_____@__/__/__
	___X_____X_____@__/__/__
	___X_____X_____@__/__/__

3

CARDIO SESSION #1

TIME:_____

ACTIVITY:_____

DURATION:_____LEVEL_____

DISTANCE:_____

CALORIES BURNED:_____

ACTIVITY PULSE RATE:_____bpm

RECOVERY PULSE RATE:_____bpm

DIFFERENCE:

DAILY SLEEP TRACKER

TIME TO BED:_____

TIME UP:_____

HOURS OF SLEEP:_____

COMMENTS:_____

DAILY AB TRACKER

EXERCISE	SET X REPS X WGT
1._____	___X_____X_____
2._____	___X_____X_____
3._____	___X_____X_____
4._____	___X_____X_____
5._____	___X_____X_____

FITNESS CLASS

(or any physical activity-walk, jog, squash)

START:_____FINISH:_____

TYPE:_____

INSTRUCTOR:_____

ESTIMATE OF
CALORIES BURNED:

COMMENTS:_____

CARDIO SESSION #2

TIME:_____

ACTIVITY:_____

DURATION:_____LEVEL_____

DISTANCE:_____

CALORIES BURNED:_____

ACTIVITY PULSE RATE:_____bpm

RECOVERY PULSE RATE:_____bpm

DIFFERENCE:_____

COMMENTS:_____

_____

TOTAL CALORIES
BURNED TODAY:

Daily Nutrition Tracking

NUTRITION	Points Goal	CAL *option*	PROT *grams*	FAT *grams*	CARB *grams*
Meal #1 – Time: H₂O_____Cups(L)					
Meal #2 – Time: H₂O_____Cups(L)					
Meal #3 – Time: H₂O_____Cups(L)					
Meal #4 – Time: H₂O_____Cups(L)					
Meal #5 – Time: H₂O_____Cups(L)					
Meal #6 – Time: H₂O_____Cups(L)					

Food Point Total For Today:

Difference (Goal Points Minus Actual Points)

3

Daily Totals: *(Add up each nutrient column. Convert each to calories. Add all and enter in "Total Calories")*   g   g   g

Conversion To Calories
Multiply Total Grams of **Pro X 4** = Calories
Multiply Total Grams of **Carb X 4**=Calories
Multiply Total Grams of **Fat X 9** = Calories

Total Calories   cal   cal   cal

Daily Percentages: (Divide total calories of each nutrient by the Total Number of Calories)   %   %   %

Total Calories Consumed:_____
            VS   **Difference**
Total Calories Burned: _____

Personal Training Log

WEIGHT TRAINING

Date:_____ Phase:_____

Start:_____ Finish:_____ Duration:_____

Day:_____ Warm Up:_____

EXERCISE	SET X REPS X WEIGHT @ TEMPO
1.	___X___X_____@__/__/__
	___X___X_____@__/__/__
	___X___X_____@__/__/__
	___X___X_____@__/__/__
	___X___X_____@__/__/__
2.	___X___X_____@__/__/__
	___X___X_____@__/__/__
	___X___X_____@__/__/__
	___X___X_____@__/__/__
	___X___X_____@__/__/__
3.	___X___X_____@__/__/__
	___X___X_____@__/__/__
	___X___X_____@__/__/__
	___X___X_____@__/__/__
	___X___X_____@__/__/__
4.	___X___X_____@__/__/__
	___X___X_____@__/__/__
	___X___X_____@__/__/__
	___X___X_____@__/__/__
	___X___X_____@__/__/__
5.	___X___X_____@__/__/__
	___X___X_____@__/__/__
	___X___X_____@__/__/__
	___X___X_____@__/__/__
	___X___X_____@__/__/__
6.	___X___X_____@__/__/__
	___X___X_____@__/__/__
	___X___X_____@__/__/__
	___X___X_____@__/__/__
	___X___X_____@__/__/__
7.	___X___X_____@__/__/__
	___X___X_____@__/__/__
	___X___X_____@__/__/__
	___X___X_____@__/__/__
	___X___X_____@__/__/__
8.	___X___X_____@__/__/__
	___X___X_____@__/__/__
	___X___X_____@__/__/__
	___X___X_____@__/__/__
	___X___X_____@__/__/__
9.	___X___X_____@__/__/__
	___X___X_____@__/__/__
	___X___X_____@__/__/__
	___X___X_____@__/__/__
	___X___X_____@__/__/__

CARDIO SESSION #1

TIME:_____

ACTIVITY:_____

DURATION:_____ LEVEL_____

DISTANCE:_____

CALORIES BURNED:_____

ACTIVITY PULSE RATE:_____bpm

RECOVERY PULSE RATE:_____bpm

DIFFERENCE:

DAILY SLEEP TRACKER

TIME TO BED:_____

TIME UP:_____

HOURS OF SLEEP:_____

COMMENTS:_____

DAILY AB TRACKER

EXERCISE	SET X REPS X WGT
1._____	___X___X___
2._____	___X___X___
3._____	___X___X___
4._____	___X___X___
5._____	___X___X___

FITNESS CLASS
(or any physical activity-walk, jog, squash)

START:_____ FINISH:_____

TYPE:_____

INSTRUCTOR:_____

ESTIMATE OF
CALORIES BURNED:

COMMENTS:_____

CARDIO SESSION #2

TIME:_____

ACTIVITY:_____

DURATION:_____ LEVEL_____

DISTANCE:_____

CALORIES BURNED:_____

ACTIVITY PULSE RATE:_____bpm

RECOVERY PULSE RATE:_____bpm

DIFFERENCE:_____

COMMENTS:_____

TOTAL CALORIES
BURNED TODAY:

NUTRITION		Points Goal	CAL *option*	PROT *grams*	FAT *grams*	CARB *grams*
Meal #1 – Time:	H$_2$O_____Cups(L)					
Meal #2 – Time:	H$_2$O_____Cups(L)					
Meal #3 – Time:	H$_2$O_____Cups(L)					
Meal #4 – Time:	H$_2$O_____Cups(L)					
Meal #5 – Time:	H$_2$O_____Cups(L)					
Meal #6 – Time:	H$_2$O_____Cups(L)					

Food Point Total For Today:					
Difference (Goal Points Minus Actual Points)					
Daily Totals: *(Add up each nutrient column. Convert each to calories. Add all and enter in "Total Calories")*			**g**	**g**	**g**
Conversion To Calories *Multiply Total Grams of **Pro** X 4 = Calories* *Multiply Total Grams of **Carb** X 4=Calories* *Multiply Total Grams of **Fat** X 9 = Calories*	***Total Calories***		**cal**	**cal**	**cal**
Daily Percentages: *(Divide total calories of each nutrient by the Total Number of Calories)*			__ %	__ %	__ %

3

***Total Calories Consumed:**_____*
 VS **Difference**
***Total Calories Burned:** _____*

Personal Training Log

WEIGHT TRAINING

Date:_____ Phase:_____

Start:_____ Finish:_____ Duration:_____

Day:_____ Warm Up:_____

EXERCISE	SET X REPS X WEIGHT @ TEMPO
1.	____X____X_____@___/__/__
	____X____X_____@___/__/__
	____X____X_____@___/__/__
	____X____X_____@___/__/__
	____X____X_____@___/__/__
2.	____X____X_____@___/__/__
	____X____X_____@___/__/__
	____X____X_____@___/__/__
	____X____X_____@___/__/__
	____X____X_____@___/__/__
3.	____X____X_____@___/__/__
	____X____X_____@___/__/__
	____X____X_____@___/__/__
	____X____X_____@___/__/__
	____X____X_____@___/__/__
4.	____X____X_____@___/__/__
	____X____X_____@___/__/__
	____X____X_____@___/__/__
	____X____X_____@___/__/__
	____X____X_____@___/__/__
5.	____X____X_____@___/__/__
	____X____X_____@___/__/__
	____X____X_____@___/__/__
	____X____X_____@___/__/__
	____X____X_____@___/__/__
6.	____X____X_____@___/__/__
	____X____X_____@___/__/__
	____X____X_____@___/__/__
	____X____X_____@___/__/__
	____X____X_____@___/__/__
7.	____X____X_____@___/__/__
	____X____X_____@___/__/__
	____X____X_____@___/__/__
	____X____X_____@___/__/__
	____X____X_____@___/__/__
8.	____X____X_____@___/__/__
	____X____X_____@___/__/__
	____X____X_____@___/__/__
	____X____X_____@___/__/__
	____X____X_____@___/__/__
9.	____X____X_____@___/__/__
	____X____X_____@___/__/__
	____X____X_____@___/__/__
	____X____X_____@___/__/__
	____X____X_____@___/__/__

3

CARDIO SESSION #1

TIME:_____

ACTIVITY:_____

DURATION:_____ LEVEL_____

DISTANCE:_____

CALORIES BURNED:_____

ACTIVITY PULSE RATE:_____ bpm

RECOVERY PULSE RATE:_____ bpm

DIFFERENCE:

DAILY SLEEP TRACKER

TIME TO BED:_____

TIME UP:_____

HOURS OF SLEEP:_____

COMMENTS:_____

DAILY AB TRACKER

EXERCISE	SET X REPS X WGT
1._____	____X____X_____
2._____	____X____X_____
3._____	____X____X_____
4._____	____X____X_____
5._____	____X____X_____

FITNESS CLASS

(or any physical activity-walk, jog, squash)

START:_____ FINISH:_____

TYPE:_____

INSTRUCTOR:_____

ESTIMATE OF
CALORIES BURNED:

COMMENTS:_____

CARDIO SESSION #2

TIME:_____

ACTIVITY:_____

DURATION:_____ LEVEL_____

DISTANCE:_____

CALORIES BURNED:_____

ACTIVITY PULSE RATE:_____ bpm

RECOVERY PULSE RATE:_____ bpm

DIFFERENCE:

COMMENTS:_____

TOTAL CALORIES
BURNED TODAY:

Daily Nutrition Tracking

NUTRITION	Points Goal	CAL *option*	PROT *grams*	FAT *grams*	CARB *grams*
Meal #1 – Time: H₂O____Cups(L)					
Meal #2 – Time: H₂O____Cups(L)					
Meal #3 – Time: H₂O____Cups(L)					
Meal #4 – Time: H₂O____Cups(L)					
Meal #5 – Time: H₂O____Cups(L)					
Meal #6 – Time: H₂O____Cups(L)					

Food Point Total For Today:					
Difference (Goal Points Minus Actual Points)					
Daily Totals: *(Add up each nutrient column. Convert each to calories. Add all and enter in "Total Calories")*			*g*	*g*	*g*
Conversion To Calories Multiply Total Grams of **Pro X 4** = Calories / Multiply Total Grams of **Carb X 4**=Calories / Multiply Total Grams of **Fat X 9** = Calories	**Total Calories**		*cal*	*cal*	*cal*
Daily Percentages: (Divide total calories of each nutrient by the Total Number of Calories)			___ *%*	___ *%*	___ *%*

Total Calories Consumed:_____

VS   **Difference**

Total Calories Burned: _____

3

Personal Training Log

WEIGHT TRAINING

Date:_____ Phase:_____
Start:_____ Finish:_____ Duration:_____
Day:_____ Warm Up:_____

EXERCISE	SET X REPS X WEIGHT @ TEMPO
1.	___X____X____ @__/__/__
	___X____X____ @__/__/__
	___X____X____ @__/__/__
	___X____X____ @__/__/__
	___X____X____ @__/__/__
2.	___X____X____ @__/__/__
	___X____X____ @__/__/__
	___X____X____ @__/__/__
	___X____X____ @__/__/__
	___X____X____ @__/__/__
3.	___X____X____ @__/__/__
	___X____X____ @__/__/__
	___X____X____ @__/__/__
	___X____X____ @__/__/__
	___X____X____ @__/__/__
4.	___X____X____ @__/__/__
	___X____X____ @__/__/__
	___X____X____ @__/__/__
	___X____X____ @__/__/__
	___X____X____ @__/__/__
5.	___X____X____ @__/__/__
	___X____X____ @__/__/__
	___X____X____ @__/__/__
	___X____X____ @__/__/__
	___X____X____ @__/__/__
6.	___X____X____ @__/__/__
	___X____X____ @__/__/__
	___X____X____ @__/__/__
	___X____X____ @__/__/__
	___X____X____ @__/__/__
7.	___X____X____ @__/__/__
	___X____X____ @__/__/__
	___X____X____ @__/__/__
	___X____X____ @__/__/__
	___X____X____ @__/__/__
8.	___X____X____ @__/__/__
	___X____X____ @__/__/__
	___X____X____ @__/__/__
	___X____X____ @__/__/__
	___X____X____ @__/__/__
9.	___X____X____ @__/__/__
	___X____X____ @__/__/__
	___X____X____ @__/__/__
	___X____X____ @__/__/__
	___X____X____ @__/__/__

CARDIO SESSION #1

TIME:_____
ACTIVITY:_____
DURATION:_____ LEVEL_____
DISTANCE:_____
CALORIES BURNED:_____
ACTIVITY PULSE RATE:_____bpm
RECOVERY PULSE RATE:_____bpm
DIFFERENCE:

DAILY SLEEP TRACKER

TIME TO BED:_____
TIME UP:_____
HOURS OF SLEEP:_____
COMMENTS:_____

DAILY AB TRACKER

EXERCISE	SET X REPS X WGT
1._____	___X____X____
2._____	___X____X____
3._____	___X____X____
4._____	___X____X____
5._____	___X____X____

FITNESS CLASS
(or any physical activity-walk, jog, squash)

START:_____ FINISH:_____
TYPE:_____
INSTRUCTOR:_____
ESTIMATE OF
CALORIES BURNED:
COMMENTS:_____

CARDIO SESSION #2

TIME:_____
ACTIVITY:_____
DURATION:_____ LEVEL_____
DISTANCE:_____
CALORIES BURNED:_____
ACTIVITY PULSE RATE:_____bpm
RECOVERY PULSE RATE:_____bpm
DIFFERENCE:_____

COMMENTS:_____

TOTAL CALORIES
BURNED TODAY:

3

Daily Nutrition Tracking

NUTRITION	Points Goal	CAL option	PROT grams	FAT grams	CARB grams
Meal #1 – Time: H₂O____Cups(L)					
Meal #2 – Time: H₂O____Cups(L)					
Meal #3 – Time: H₂O____Cups(L)					
Meal #4 – Time: H₂O____Cups(L)					
Meal #5 – Time: H₂O____Cups(L)					
Meal #6 – Time: H₂O____Cups(L)					

Food Point Total For Today:		
Difference (Goal Points Minus Actual Points)		

Daily Totals: (Add up each nutrient column. Convert each to calories. Add all and enter in "Total Calories") | g | g | g |

Conversion To Calories
Multiply Total Grams of **Pro X 4** = Calories
Multiply Total Grams of **Carb X 4**=Calories
Multiply Total Grams of **Fat X 9** = Calories | **Total Calories** | cal | cal | cal |

Daily Percentages: (Divide total calories of each nutrient by the Total Number of Calories) | % | % | % |

Total Calories Consumed:_____
               VS   **Difference**
Total Calories Burned: _____

3

Personal Training Log

WEIGHT TRAINING	CARDIO SESSION #1

WEIGHT TRAINING

Date:_____ Phase:_____

Start:_____ Finish:_____ Duration:_____

Day:_____ Warm Up:_____

EXERCISE	SET X REPS X WEIGHT @ TEMPO
1.	___X___X_____@__/__/__
	___X___X_____@__/__/__
	___X___X_____@__/__/__
	___X___X_____@__/__/__
	___X___X_____@__/__/__
2.	___X___X_____@__/__/__
	___X___X_____@__/__/__
	___X___X_____@__/__/__
	___X___X_____@__/__/__
	___X___X_____@__/__/__
3.	___X___X_____@__/__/__
	___X___X_____@__/__/__
	___X___X_____@__/__/__
	___X___X_____@__/__/__
	___X___X_____@__/__/__
4.	___X___X_____@__/__/__
	___X___X_____@__/__/__
	___X___X_____@__/__/__
	___X___X_____@__/__/__
	___X___X_____@__/__/__
5.	___X___X_____@__/__/__
	___X___X_____@__/__/__
	___X___X_____@__/__/__
	___X___X_____@__/__/__
	___X___X_____@__/__/__
6.	___X___X_____@__/__/__
	___X___X_____@__/__/__
	___X___X_____@__/__/__
	___X___X_____@__/__/__
	___X___X_____@__/__/__
7.	___X___X_____@__/__/__
	___X___X_____@__/__/__
	___X___X_____@__/__/__
	___X___X_____@__/__/__
	___X___X_____@__/__/__
8.	___X___X_____@__/__/__
	___X___X_____@__/__/__
	___X___X_____@__/__/__
	___X___X_____@__/__/__
	___X___X_____@__/__/__
9.	___X___X_____@__/__/__
	___X___X_____@__/__/__
	___X___X_____@__/__/__
	___X___X_____@__/__/__
	___X___X_____@__/__/__

CARDIO SESSION #1

TIME:_____

ACTIVITY:_____

DURATION:_____ LEVEL_____

DISTANCE:_____

CALORIES BURNED:_____

ACTIVITY PULSE RATE:_____ bpm

RECOVERY PULSE RATE:_____ bpm

DIFFERENCE:

DAILY SLEEP TRACKER

TIME TO BED:_____

TIME UP:_____

HOURS OF SLEEP:_____

COMMENTS:_____

DAILY AB TRACKER

EXERCISE	SET X REPS X WGT
1._____	___X___X___
2._____	___X___X___
3._____	___X___X___
4._____	___X___X___
5._____	___X___X___

FITNESS CLASS
(or any physical activity-walk, jog, squash)

START:_____ FINISH:_____

TYPE:_____

INSTRUCTOR:_____

ESTIMATE OF
CALORIES BURNED: [_____]

COMMENTS:_____

CARDIO SESSION #2

TIME:_____

ACTIVITY:_____

DURATION:_____ LEVEL_____

DISTANCE:_____

CALORIES BURNED:_____

ACTIVITY PULSE RATE:_____ bpm

RECOVERY PULSE RATE:_____ bpm

DIFFERENCE:_____

COMMENTS:_____

TOTAL CALORIES
BURNED TODAY: [_____]

NUTRITION	Points Goal	CAL *option*	PROT *grams*	FAT *grams*	CARB *grams*
Meal #1 – Time: H₂O____Cups(L)					
Meal #2 – Time: H₂O____Cups(L)					
Meal #3 – Time: H₂O____Cups(L)					
Meal #4 – Time: H₂O____Cups(L)					
Meal #5 – Time: H₂O____Cups(L)					
Meal #6 – Time: H₂O____Cups(L)					

Food Point Total For Today:

Difference (Goal Points Minus Actual Points)

Daily Totals: (Add up each nutrient column. Convert each to calories. Add all and enter in "Total Calories")   g   g   g

Conversion To Calories
Multiply Total Grams of **Pro X 4** = Calories
Multiply Total Grams of **Carb X 4** = Calories
Multiply Total Grams of **Fat X 9** = Calories

Total Calories   cal   cal   cal

Daily Percentages: (Divide total calories of each nutrient by the Total Number of Calories)   %   %   %

Total Calories Consumed:_____
VS   **Difference**
Total Calories Burned: _____

3

Personal Training Log

WEIGHT TRAINING

Date:_____ Phase:_____

Start:_____ Finish:_____ Duration:_____

Day:_____ Warm Up:_____

EXERCISE	SET X REPS X WEIGHT @ TEMPO
1.	___X___X_____@__/__/__
	___X___X_____@__/__/__
	___X___X_____@__/__/__
	___X___X_____@__/__/__
	___X___X_____@__/__/__
2.	___X___X_____@__/__/__
	___X___X_____@__/__/__
	___X___X_____@__/__/__
	___X___X_____@__/__/__
	___X___X_____@__/__/__
3.	___X___X_____@__/__/__
	___X___X_____@__/__/__
	___X___X_____@__/__/__
	___X___X_____@__/__/__
	___X___X_____@__/__/__
4.	___X___X_____@__/__/__
	___X___X_____@__/__/__
	___X___X_____@__/__/__
	___X___X_____@__/__/__
	___X___X_____@__/__/__
5.	___X___X_____@__/__/__
	___X___X_____@__/__/__
	___X___X_____@__/__/__
	___X___X_____@__/__/__
	___X___X_____@__/__/__
6.	___X___X_____@__/__/__
	___X___X_____@__/__/__
	___X___X_____@__/__/__
	___X___X_____@__/__/__
	___X___X_____@__/__/__
7.	___X___X_____@__/__/__
	___X___X_____@__/__/__
	___X___X_____@__/__/__
	___X___X_____@__/__/__
	___X___X_____@__/__/__
8.	___X___X_____@__/__/__
	___X___X_____@__/__/__
	___X___X_____@__/__/__
	___X___X_____@__/__/__
	___X___X_____@__/__/__
9.	___X___X_____@__/__/__
	___X___X_____@__/__/__
	___X___X_____@__/__/__
	___X___X_____@__/__/__
	___X___X_____@__/__/__

CARDIO SESSION #1

TIME:_____

ACTIVITY:_____

DURATION:_____ LEVEL_____

DISTANCE:_____

CALORIES BURNED:_____

ACTIVITY PULSE RATE:_____bpm

RECOVERY PULSE RATE:_____bpm

DIFFERENCE:

DAILY SLEEP TRACKER

TIME TO BED:_____

TIME UP:_____

HOURS OF SLEEP:_____

COMMENTS:_____

DAILY AB TRACKER

EXERCISE	SET X REPS X WGT
1._____	___X___X___
2._____	___X___X___
3._____	___X___X___
4._____	___X___X___
5._____	___X___X___

FITNESS CLASS

(or any physical activity-walk, jog, squash)

START:_____ FINISH:_____

TYPE:_____

INSTRUCTOR:_____

ESTIMATE OF
CALORIES BURNED:

COMMENTS:_____

CARDIO SESSION #2

TIME:_____

ACTIVITY:_____

DURATION:_____ LEVEL_____

DISTANCE:_____

CALORIES BURNED:_____

ACTIVITY PULSE RATE:_____bpm

RECOVERY PULSE RATE:_____bpm

DIFFERENCE:_____

COMMENTS:_____

TOTAL CALORIES
BURNED TODAY:

NUTRITION	Points Goal	CAL *option*	PROT *grams*	FAT *grams*	CARB *grams*
Meal #1 – Time: H₂O_____Cups(L)					
Meal #2 – Time: H₂O_____Cups(L)					
Meal #3 – Time: H₂O_____Cups(L)					
Meal #4 – Time: H₂O_____Cups(L)					
Meal #5 – Time: H₂O_____Cups(L)					
Meal #6 – Time: H₂O_____Cups(L)					

Food Point Total For Today:

Difference (Goal Points Minus Actual Points)

3

Daily Totals: *(Add up each nutrient column. Convert each to calories. Add all and enter in "Total Calories")*   g   g   g

Conversion To Calories
*Multiply Total Grams of **Pro** X 4 = Calories*
*Multiply Total Grams of **Carb** X 4 = Calories*
*Multiply Total Grams of **Fat** X 9 = Calories*

Total Calories   cal   cal   cal

Daily Percentages: (*Divide total calories of each nutrient by the Total Number of Calories*)   ___%   ___%   ___%

Total Calories Consumed:_____
        VS   **Difference**
Total Calories Burned: _____

Personal Training Log

WEIGHT TRAINING

Date:_____ Phase:_____

Start:_____ Finish:_____ Duration:_____

Day:_____ Warm Up:_____

EXERCISE	SET X REPS X WEIGHT @ TEMPO
1.	___X___X___ @__/__/__
	___X___X___ @__/__/__
	___X___X___ @__/__/__
	___X___X___ @__/__/__
	___X___X___ @__/__/__
2.	___X___X___ @__/__/__
	___X___X___ @__/__/__
	___X___X___ @__/__/__
	___X___X___ @__/__/__
	___X___X___ @__/__/__
3.	___X___X___ @__/__/__
	___X___X___ @__/__/__
	___X___X___ @__/__/__
	___X___X___ @__/__/__
	___X___X___ @__/__/__
4.	___X___X___ @__/__/__
	___X___X___ @__/__/__
	___X___X___ @__/__/__
	___X___X___ @__/__/__
	___X___X___ @__/__/__
5.	___X___X___ @__/__/__
	___X___X___ @__/__/__
	___X___X___ @__/__/__
	___X___X___ @__/__/__
	___X___X___ @__/__/__
6.	___X___X___ @__/__/__
	___X___X___ @__/__/__
	___X___X___ @__/__/__
	___X___X___ @__/__/__
	___X___X___ @__/__/__
7.	___X___X___ @__/__/__
	___X___X___ @__/__/__
	___X___X___ @__/__/__
	___X___X___ @__/__/__
	___X___X___ @__/__/__
8.	___X___X___ @__/__/__
	___X___X___ @__/__/__
	___X___X___ @__/__/__
	___X___X___ @__/__/__
	___X___X___ @__/__/__
9.	___X___X___ @__/__/__
	___X___X___ @__/__/__
	___X___X___ @__/__/__
	___X___X___ @__/__/__
	___X___X___ @__/__/__

CARDIO SESSION #1

TIME:_____

ACTIVITY:_____

DURATION:_____ LEVEL_____

DISTANCE:_____

CALORIES BURNED:_____

ACTIVITY PULSE RATE:_____bpm

RECOVERY PULSE RATE:_____bpm

DIFFERENCE:_____

DAILY SLEEP TRACKER

TIME TO BED:_____

TIME UP:_____

HOURS OF SLEEP:_____

COMMENTS:_____

DAILY AB TRACKER

EXERCISE	SET X REPS X WGT
1._____	___X___X___
2._____	___X___X___
3._____	___X___X___
4._____	___X___X___
5._____	___X___X___

FITNESS CLASS
(or any physical activity-walk, jog, squash)

START:_____ FINISH:_____

TYPE:_____

INSTRUCTOR:_____

ESTIMATE OF
CALORIES BURNED:

COMMENTS:_____

CARDIO SESSION #2

TIME:_____

ACTIVITY:_____

DURATION:_____ LEVEL_____

DISTANCE:_____

CALORIES BURNED:_____

ACTIVITY PULSE RATE:_____bpm

RECOVERY PULSE RATE:_____bpm

DIFFERENCE:_____

COMMENTS:_____

TOTAL CALORIES
BURNED TODAY:

Daily Nutrition Tracking

NUTRITION	Points Goal	CAL *option*	PROT *grams*	FAT *grams*	CARB *grams*
Meal #1 – Time: H₂O____Cups(L)					
Meal #2 – Time: H₂O____Cups(L)					
Meal #3 – Time: H₂O____Cups(L)					
Meal #4 – Time: H₂O____Cups(L)					
Meal #5 – Time: H₂O____Cups(L)					
Meal #6 – Time: H₂O____Cups(L)					

Food Point Total For Today:					
Difference (Goal Points Minus Actual Points)					
Daily Totals: *(Add up each nutrient column. Convert each to calories. Add all and enter in "Total Calories")*			*g*	*g*	*g*
Conversion To Calories — Multiply Total Grams of **Pro X 4** = Calories; Multiply Total Grams of **Carb X 4**=Calories; Multiply Total Grams of **Fat X 9** = Calories	**Total Calories**		*cal*	*cal*	*cal*
Daily Percentages: (Divide total calories of each nutrient by the Total Number of Calories)			__ *%*	__ *%*	__ *%*

3

Total Calories Consumed:_____
 VS   ***Difference***
Total Calories Burned: _____

Personal Training Log

WEIGHT TRAINING

Date:_____ Phase:_____

Start:_____ Finish:_____ Duration:_____

Day:_____ Warm Up:_____

EXERCISE	SET X REPS X WEIGHT @ TEMPO
1.	___X___ X _____ @__/__/__
	___X___ X _____ @__/__/__
	___X___ X _____ @__/__/__
	___X___ X _____ @__/__/__
	___X___ X _____ @__/__/__
2.	___X___ X _____ @__/__/__
	___X___ X _____ @__/__/__
	___X___ X _____ @__/__/__
	___X___ X _____ @__/__/__
	___X___ X _____ @__/__/__
3.	___X___ X _____ @__/__/__
	___X___ X _____ @__/__/__
	___X___ X _____ @__/__/__
	___X___ X _____ @__/__/__
	___X___ X _____ @__/__/__
4.	___X___ X _____ @__/__/__
	___X___ X _____ @__/__/__
	___X___ X _____ @__/__/__
	___X___ X _____ @__/__/__
	___X___ X _____ @__/__/__
5.	___X___ X _____ @__/__/__
	___X___ X _____ @__/__/__
	___X___ X _____ @__/__/__
	___X___ X _____ @__/__/__
	___X___ X _____ @__/__/__
6.	___X___ X _____ @__/__/__
	___X___ X _____ @__/__/__
	___X___ X _____ @__/__/__
	___X___ X _____ @__/__/__
	___X___ X _____ @__/__/__
7.	___X___ X _____ @__/__/__
	___X___ X _____ @__/__/__
	___X___ X _____ @__/__/__
	___X___ X _____ @__/__/__
	___X___ X _____ @__/__/__
8.	___X___ X _____ @__/__/__
	___X___ X _____ @__/__/__
	___X___ X _____ @__/__/__
	___X___ X _____ @__/__/__
	___X___ X _____ @__/__/__
9.	___X___ X _____ @__/__/__
	___X___ X _____ @__/__/__
	___X___ X _____ @__/__/__
	___X___ X _____ @__/__/__
	___X___ X _____ @__/__/__

CARDIO SESSION #1

TIME:_____

ACTIVITY:_____

DURATION:_____ LEVEL_____

DISTANCE:_____

CALORIES BURNED:_____

ACTIVITY PULSE RATE:_____ bpm

RECOVERY PULSE RATE:_____ bpm

DIFFERENCE:

DAILY SLEEP TRACKER

TIME TO BED:_____

TIME UP:_____

HOURS OF SLEEP:_____

COMMENTS:_____

DAILY AB TRACKER

EXERCISE	SET X REPS X WGT
1._____	___X___ X___
2._____	___X___ X___
3._____	___X___ X___
4._____	___X___ X___
5._____	___X___ X___

FITNESS CLASS

(or any physical activity-walk, jog, squash)

START:_____ FINISH:_____

TYPE:_____

INSTRUCTOR:_____

ESTIMATE OF
CALORIES BURNED: [ ]

COMMENTS:_____

CARDIO SESSION #2

TIME:_____

ACTIVITY:_____

DURATION:_____ LEVEL_____

DISTANCE:_____

CALORIES BURNED:_____

ACTIVITY PULSE RATE:_____ bpm

RECOVERY PULSE RATE:_____ bpm

DIFFERENCE: _____

COMMENTS:_____

TOTAL CALORIES
BURNED TODAY: [ ]

NUTRITION	Points Goal	CAL *option*	PROT *grams*	FAT *grams*	CARB *grams*
Meal #1 – Time: H₂O_____Cups(L)					
Meal #2 – Time: H₂O_____Cups(L)					
Meal #3 – Time: H₂O_____Cups(L)					
Meal #4 – Time: H₂O_____Cups(L)					
Meal #5 – Time: H₂O_____Cups(L)					
Meal #6 – Time: H₂O_____Cups(L)					
Food Point Total For Today:					
Difference (Goal Points Minus Actual Points)					
Daily Totals: *(Add up each nutrient column. Convert each to calories. Add all and enter in "Total Calories")*			*g*	*g*	*g*

Conversion To Calories *Multiply Total Grams of* **Pro X 4** *= Calories* *Multiply Total Grams of* **Carb X 4** *=Calories* *Multiply Total Grams of* **Fat X 9** *= Calories*	***Total Calories***	*cal*	*cal*	*cal*

Daily Percentages: (*Divide total calories of each nutrient by the Total Number of Calories*)	____ *%*	____ *%*	____ *%*

Total Calories Consumed:_____
VS   **Difference**
Total Calories Burned: _____

3

Personal Training Log

WEIGHT TRAINING

Date:_____ Phase:_____

Start:_____ Finish:_____ Duration:_____

Day:_____ Warm Up:_____

EXERCISE	SET X REPS X WEIGHT @ TEMPO
1.	___X___ X_____ @___ /__ /__
	___X___ X_____ @___ /__ /__
	___X___ X_____ @___ /__ /__
	___X___ X_____ @___ /__ /__
	___X___ X_____ @___ /__ /__
2.	___X___ X_____ @___ /__ /__
	___X___ X_____ @___ /__ /__
	___X___ X_____ @___ /__ /__
	___X___ X_____ @___ /__ /__
	___X___ X_____ @___ /__ /__
3.	___X___ X_____ @___ /__ /__
	___X___ X_____ @___ /__ /__
	___X___ X_____ @___ /__ /__
	___X___ X_____ @___ /__ /__
	___X___ X_____ @___ /__ /__
4.	___X___ X_____ @___ /__ /__
	___X___ X_____ @___ /__ /__
	___X___ X_____ @___ /__ /__
	___X___ X_____ @___ /__ /__
	___X___ X_____ @___ /__ /__
5.	___X___ X_____ @___ /__ /__
	___X___ X_____ @___ /__ /__
	___X___ X_____ @___ /__ /__
	___X___ X_____ @___ /__ /__
	___X___ X_____ @___ /__ /__
6.	___X___ X_____ @___ /__ /__
	___X___ X_____ @___ /__ /__
	___X___ X_____ @___ /__ /__
	___X___ X_____ @___ /__ /__
	___X___ X_____ @___ /__ /__
7.	___X___ X_____ @___ /__ /__
	___X___ X_____ @___ /__ /__
	___X___ X_____ @___ /__ /__
	___X___ X_____ @___ /__ /__
	___X___ X_____ @___ /__ /__
8.	___X___ X_____ @___ /__ /__
	___X___ X_____ @___ /__ /__
	___X___ X_____ @___ /__ /__
	___X___ X_____ @___ /__ /__
	___X___ X_____ @___ /__ /__
9.	___X___ X_____ @___ /__ /__
	___X___ X_____ @___ /__ /__
	___X___ X_____ @___ /__ /__
	___X___ X_____ @___ /__ /__
	___X___ X_____ @___ /__ /__

CARDIO SESSION #1

TIME:_____

ACTIVITY:_____

DURATION:_____ LEVEL_____

DISTANCE:_____

CALORIES BURNED:_____

ACTIVITY PULSE RATE:_____bpm

RECOVERY PULSE RATE:_____bpm

DIFFERENCE:

DAILY SLEEP TRACKER

TIME TO BED:_____

TIME UP:_____

HOURS OF SLEEP:_____

COMMENTS:_____

DAILY AB TRACKER

EXERCISE	SET X REPS X WGT
1._____	___X____ X_____
2._____	___X____ X_____
3._____	___X____ X_____
4._____	___X____ X_____
5._____	___X____ X_____

FITNESS CLASS

(or any physical activity-walk, jog, squash)

START:_____ FINISH:_____

TYPE:_____

INSTRUCTOR:_____

ESTIMATE OF
CALORIES BURNED: [ ]

COMMENTS:_____

CARDIO SESSION #2

TIME:_____

ACTIVITY:_____

DURATION:_____ LEVEL_____

DISTANCE:_____

CALORIES BURNED:_____

ACTIVITY PULSE RATE:_____bpm

RECOVERY PULSE RATE:_____bpm

DIFFERENCE:_____

COMMENTS:_____

TOTAL CALORIES
BURNED TODAY: [ ]

NUTRITION	Points Goal	CAL option	PROT grams	FAT grams	CARB grams
Meal #1 – Time: H₂O____Cups(L)					
Meal #2 – Time: H₂O____Cups(L)					
Meal #3 – Time: H₂O____Cups(L)					
Meal #4 – Time: H₂O____Cups(L)					
Meal #5 – Time: H₂O____Cups(L)					
Meal #6 – Time: H₂O____Cups(L)					

Food Point Total For Today:					
Difference (Goal Points Minus Actual Points)					
Daily Totals: (Add up each nutrient column. Convert each to calories. Add all and enter in "Total Calories")			g	g	g

Conversion To Calories Multiply Total Grams of **Pro X 4** = Calories Multiply Total Grams of **Carb X 4**=Calories Multiply Total Grams of **Fat X 9** = Calories	**Total Calories**	cal	cal	cal

Daily Percentages: (Divide total calories of each nutrient by the Total Number of Calories)	%	%	%

Total Calories Consumed:_____

 VS **Difference**

Total Calories Burned: _____

3

Personal Training Log

WEIGHT TRAINING

Date:_____ Phase:_____

Start:_____ Finish:_____ Duration:_____

Day:_____ Warm Up:_____

EXERCISE	SET X REPS X WEIGHT @ TEMPO
1.	___X___X_____@__/__/__ ___X___X_____@__/__/__ ___X___X_____@__/__/__ ___X___X_____@__/__/__ ___X___X_____@__/__/__
2.	___X___X_____@__/__/__ ___X___X_____@__/__/__ ___X___X_____@__/__/__ ___X___X_____@__/__/__ ___X___X_____@__/__/__
3.	___X___X_____@__/__/__ ___X___X_____@__/__/__ ___X___X_____@__/__/__ ___X___X_____@__/__/__ ___X___X_____@__/__/__
4.	___X___X_____@__/__/__ ___X___X_____@__/__/__ ___X___X_____@__/__/__ ___X___X_____@__/__/__ ___X___X_____@__/__/__
5.	___X___X_____@__/__/__ ___X___X_____@__/__/__ ___X___X_____@__/__/__ ___X___X_____@__/__/__ ___X___X_____@__/__/__
6.	___X___X_____@__/__/__ ___X___X_____@__/__/__ ___X___X_____@__/__/__ ___X___X_____@__/__/__ ___X___X_____@__/__/__
7.	___X___X_____@__/__/__ ___X___X_____@__/__/__ ___X___X_____@__/__/__ ___X___X_____@__/__/__ ___X___X_____@__/__/__
8.	___X___X_____@__/__/__ ___X___X_____@__/__/__ ___X___X_____@__/__/__ ___X___X_____@__/__/__ ___X___X_____@__/__/__
9.	___X___X_____@__/__/__ ___X___X_____@__/__/__ ___X___X_____@__/__/__ ___X___X_____@__/__/__ ___X___X_____@__/__/__

CARDIO SESSION #1

TIME:_____

ACTIVITY:_____

DURATION:_____LEVEL_____

DISTANCE:_____

CALORIES BURNED:_____

ACTIVITY PULSE RATE:_____bpm

RECOVERY PULSE RATE:_____bpm

DIFFERENCE:

DAILY SLEEP TRACKER

TIME TO BED:_____

TIME UP:_____

HOURS OF SLEEP:_____

COMMENTS:_____

DAILY AB TRACKER

EXERCISE	SET X REPS X WGT
1._____	___X___X___
2._____	___X___X___
3._____	___X___X___
4._____	___X___X___
5._____	___X___X___

FITNESS CLASS

(or any physical activity-walk, jog, squash)

START:_____FINISH:_____

TYPE:_____

INSTRUCTOR:_____

ESTIMATE OF
CALORIES BURNED:

COMMENTS:_____

CARDIO SESSION #2

TIME:_____

ACTIVITY:_____

DURATION:_____LEVEL_____

DISTANCE:_____

CALORIES BURNED:_____

ACTIVITY PULSE RATE:_____bpm

RECOVERY PULSE RATE:_____bpm

DIFFERENCE:_____

COMMENTS:_____

_____

TOTAL CALORIES
BURNED TODAY:

Daily Nutrition Tracking

NUTRITION	Points Goal	CAL *option*	PROT *grams*	FAT *grams*	CARB *grams*
Meal #1 – Time: H₂O____Cups(L)					
Meal #2 – Time: H₂O____Cups(L)					
Meal #3 – Time: H₂O____Cups(L)					
Meal #4 – Time: H₂O____Cups(L)					
Meal #5 – Time: H₂O____Cups(L)					
Meal #6 Time: H₂O____Cups(L)					
Food Point Total For Today:					
Difference (Goal Points Minus Actual Points)					
Daily Totals:(Add up each nutrient column. Convert each to calories. Add all and enter in "Total Calories")			g	g	g
Conversion To Calories Multiply Total Grams of **Pro X 4** = Calories Multiply Total Grams of **Carb X 4**=Calories Multiply Total Grams of **Fat X 9** = Calories	***Total Calories***		cal	cal	cal
Daily Percentages: (Divide total calories of each nutrient by the Total Number of Calories)			%	%	%

Total Calories Consumed:_____
          VS   *Difference*
Total Calories Burned: _____

3

Personal Training Log

WEIGHT TRAINING

Date:_____ Phase:_____

Start:_____ Finish:_____ Duration:_____

Day:_____ Warm Up:_____

EXERCISE	SET X REPS X WEIGHT @ TEMPO
1.	___ X ___ X ___ @ __ / __ / __
	___ X ___ X ___ @ __ / __ / __
	___ X ___ X ___ @ __ / __ / __
	___ X ___ X ___ @ __ / __ / __
	___ X ___ X ___ @ __ / __ / __
2.	___ X ___ X ___ @ __ / __ / __
	___ X ___ X ___ @ __ / __ / __
	___ X ___ X ___ @ __ / __ / __
	___ X ___ X ___ @ __ / __ / __
	___ X ___ X ___ @ __ / __ / __
3.	___ X ___ X ___ @ __ / __ / __
	___ X ___ X ___ @ __ / __ / __
	___ X ___ X ___ @ __ / __ / __
	___ X ___ X ___ @ __ / __ / __
	___ X ___ X ___ @ __ / __ / __
4.	___ X ___ X ___ @ __ / __ / __
	___ X ___ X ___ @ __ / __ / __
	___ X ___ X ___ @ __ / __ / __
	___ X ___ X ___ @ __ / __ / __
	___ X ___ X ___ @ __ / __ / __
5.	___ X ___ X ___ @ __ / __ / __
	___ X ___ X ___ @ __ / __ / __
	___ X ___ X ___ @ __ / __ / __
	___ X ___ X ___ @ __ / __ / __
	___ X ___ X ___ @ __ / __ / __
6.	___ X ___ X ___ @ __ / __ / __
	___ X ___ X ___ @ __ / __ / __
	___ X ___ X ___ @ __ / __ / __
	___ X ___ X ___ @ __ / __ / __
	___ X ___ X ___ @ __ / __ / __
7.	___ X ___ X ___ @ __ / __ / __
	___ X ___ X ___ @ __ / __ / __
	___ X ___ X ___ @ __ / __ / __
	___ X ___ X ___ @ __ / __ / __
	___ X ___ X ___ @ __ / __ / __
8.	___ X ___ X ___ @ __ / __ / __
	___ X ___ X ___ @ __ / __ / __
	___ X ___ X ___ @ __ / __ / __
	___ X ___ X ___ @ __ / __ / __
	___ X ___ X ___ @ __ / __ / __
9.	___ X ___ X ___ @ __ / __ / __
	___ X ___ X ___ @ __ / __ / __
	___ X ___ X ___ @ __ / __ / __
	___ X ___ X ___ @ __ / __ / __
	___ X ___ X ___ @ __ / __ / __

CARDIO SESSION #1

TIME:_____

ACTIVITY:_____

DURATION:_____ LEVEL_____

DISTANCE:_____

CALORIES BURNED:_____

ACTIVITY PULSE RATE:_____ bpm

RECOVERY PULSE RATE:_____ bpm

DIFFERENCE:

DAILY SLEEP TRACKER

TIME TO BED:_____

TIME UP:_____

HOURS OF SLEEP:_____

COMMENTS:_____

DAILY AB TRACKER

EXERCISE	SET X REPS X WGT
1._____	___ X ___ X ___
2._____	___ X ___ X ___
3._____	___ X ___ X ___
4._____	___ X ___ X ___
5._____	___ X ___ X ___

FITNESS CLASS

(or any physical activity-walk, jog, squash)

START:_____ FINISH:_____

TYPE:_____

INSTRUCTOR:_____

ESTIMATE OF CALORIES BURNED: [____]

COMMENTS:_____

CARDIO SESSION #2

TIME:_____

ACTIVITY:_____

DURATION:_____ LEVEL_____

DISTANCE:_____

CALORIES BURNED:_____

ACTIVITY PULSE RATE:_____ bpm

RECOVERY PULSE RATE:_____ bpm

DIFFERENCE:_____

COMMENTS:_____

TOTAL CALORIES BURNED TODAY: [____]

NUTRITION	Points Goal	CAL *option*	PROT *grams*	FAT *grams*	CARB *grams*
Meal #1 – Time: H₂O____Cups(L)					
Meal #2 – Time: H₂O____Cups(L)					
Meal #3 – Time: H₂O____Cups(L)					
Meal #4 – Time: H₂O____Cups(L)					
Meal #5 – Time: H₂O____Cups(L)					
Meal #6 Time: H₂O____Cups(L)					
Food Point Total For Today:					
Difference *(Goal Points Minus Actual Points)*					
Daily Totals: *(Add up each nutrient column. Convert each to calories. Add all and enter in "Total Calories")*			*g*	*g*	*g*

Conversion To Calories Multiply Total Grams of **Pro X 4** = Calories Multiply Total Grams of **Carb X 4**=Calories Multiply Total Grams of **Fat X 9** = Calories	**Total Calories**	*cal*	*cal*	*cal*

Daily Percentages: *(Divide total calories of each nutrient by the Total Number of Calories)*	___ *%*	___ *%*	___ *%*

Total Calories Consumed:_____

            VS   **Difference**

Total Calories Burned: _____

3

Personal Training Log

WEIGHT TRAINING

Date:_____ Phase:_____

Start:_____ Finish:_____ Duration:_____

Day:_____ Warm Up:_____

EXERCISE	SET X REPS X WEIGHT @ TEMPO
1.	___X___X_____@___/___/___
	___X___X_____@___/___/___
	___X___X_____@___/___/___
	___X___X_____@___/___/___
	___X___X_____@___/___/___
2.	___X___X_____@___/___/___
	___X___X_____@___/___/___
	___X___X_____@___/___/___
	___X___X_____@___/___/___
	___X___X_____@___/___/___
3.	___X___X_____@___/___/___
	___X___X_____@___/___/___
	___X___X_____@___/___/___
	___X___X_____@___/___/___
	___X___X_____@___/___/___
4.	___X___X_____@___/___/___
	___X___X_____@___/___/___
	___X___X_____@___/___/___
	___X___X_____@___/___/___
	___X___X_____@___/___/___
5.	___X___X_____@___/___/___
	___X___X_____@___/___/___
	___X___X_____@___/___/___
	___X___X_____@___/___/___
	___X___X_____@___/___/___
6.	___X___X_____@___/___/___
	___X___X_____@___/___/___
	___X___X_____@___/___/___
	___X___X_____@___/___/___
	___X___X_____@___/___/___
7.	___X___X_____@___/___/___
	___X___X_____@___/___/___
	___X___X_____@___/___/___
	___X___X_____@___/___/___
	___X___X_____@___/___/___
8.	___X___X_____@___/___/___
	___X___X_____@___/___/___
	___X___X_____@___/___/___
	___X___X_____@___/___/___
	___X___X_____@___/___/___
9.	___X___X_____@___/___/___
	___X___X_____@___/___/___
	___X___X_____@___/___/___
	___X___X_____@___/___/___
	___X___X_____@___/___/___

CARDIO SESSION #1

TIME:_____

ACTIVITY:_____

DURATION:_____ LEVEL_____

DISTANCE:_____

CALORIES BURNED:_____

ACTIVITY PULSE RATE:_____bpm

RECOVERY PULSE RATE:_____bpm

DIFFERENCE:

DAILY SLEEP TRACKER

TIME TO BED:_____

TIME UP:_____

HOURS OF SLEEP:_____

COMMENTS:_____

DAILY AB TRACKER

EXERCISE	SET X REPS X WGT
1._____	___X___X___
2._____	___X___X___
3._____	___X___X___
4._____	___X___X___
5._____	___X___X___

FITNESS CLASS

(or any physical activity-walk, jog, squash)

START:_____ FINISH:_____

TYPE:_____

INSTRUCTOR:_____

ESTIMATE OF
CALORIES BURNED:

COMMENTS:_____

CARDIO SESSION #2

TIME:_____

ACTIVITY:_____

DURATION:_____ LEVEL_____

DISTANCE:_____

CALORIES BURNED:_____

ACTIVITY PULSE RATE:_____bpm

RECOVERY PULSE RATE:_____bpm

DIFFERENCE:_____

COMMENTS:_____

TOTAL CALORIES
BURNED TODAY:

3

NUTRITION	Points Goal	CAL *option*	PROT *grams*	FAT *grams*	CARB *grams*
Meal #1 – Time: H₂O_____Cups(L)					
Meal #2 – Time: H₂O_____Cups(L)					
Meal #3 – Time: H₂O_____Cups(L)					
Meal #4 – Time: H₂O_____Cups(L)					
Meal #5 – Time: H₂O_____Cups(L)					
Meal #6 – Time: H₂O_____Cups(L)					

Food Point Total For Today:					
Difference (Goal Points Minus Actual Points)					
Daily Totals: (Add up each nutrient column. Convert each to calories. Add all and enter in "Total Calories")			g	g	g
Conversion To Calories Multiply Total Grams of **Pro X 4** = Calories / Multiply Total Grams of **Carb X 4** =Calories / Multiply Total Grams of **Fat X 9** = Calories	**Total Calories**		cal	cal	cal
Daily Percentages: (Divide total calories of each nutrient by the Total Number of Calories)			___ %	___ %	___ %

3

Total Calories Consumed:_____
                    VS   **Difference**
Total Calories Burned: _____

Personal Training Log

WEIGHT TRAINING

Date:_____Phase:_____

Start:_____Finish:_____Duration:_____

Day:_____Warm Up:_____

EXERCISE	SET X REPS X WEIGHT @ TEMPO
1.	___X_____X_____@__/__/__
	___X_____X_____@__/__/__
	___X_____X_____@__/__/__
	___X_____X_____@__/__/__
	___X_____X_____@__/__/__
2.	___X_____X_____@__/__/__
	___X_____X_____@__/__/__
	___X_____X_____@__/__/__
	___X_____X_____@__/__/__
	___X_____X_____@__/__/__
3.	___X_____X_____@__/__/__
	___X_____X_____@__/__/__
	___X_____X_____@__/__/__
	___X_____X_____@__/__/__
	___X_____X_____@__/__/__
4.	___X_____X_____@__/__/__
	___X_____X_____@__/__/__
	___X_____X_____@__/__/__
	___X_____X_____@__/__/__
	___X_____X_____@__/__/__
5.	___X_____X_____@__/__/__
	___X_____X_____@__/__/__
	___X_____X_____@__/__/__
	___X_____X_____@__/__/__
	___X_____X_____@__/__/__
6.	___X_____X_____@__/__/__
	___X_____X_____@__/__/__
	___X_____X_____@__/__/__
	___X_____X_____@__/__/__
	___X_____X_____@__/__/__
7.	___X_____X_____@__/__/__
	___X_____X_____@__/__/__
	___X_____X_____@__/__/__
	___X_____X_____@__/__/__
	___X_____X_____@__/__/__
8.	___X_____X_____@__/__/__
	___X_____X_____@__/__/__
	___X_____X_____@__/__/__
	___X_____X_____@__/__/__
	___X_____X_____@__/__/__
9.	___X_____X_____@__/__/__
	___X_____X_____@__/__/__
	___X_____X_____@__/__/__
	___X_____X_____@__/__/__
	___X_____X_____@__/__/__

CARDIO SESSION #1

TIME:_____

ACTIVITY:_____

DURATION:_____LEVEL_____

DISTANCE:_____

CALORIES BURNED:_____

ACTIVITY PULSE RATE:_____bpm

RECOVERY PULSE RATE:_____bpm

DIFFERENCE:

DAILY SLEEP TRACKER

TIME TO BED:_____

TIME UP:_____

HOURS OF SLEEP:_____

COMMENTS:_____

DAILY AB TRACKER

EXERCISE	SET X REPS X WGT
1._____	___X_____X_____
2._____	___X_____X_____
3._____	___X_____X_____
4._____	___X_____X_____
5._____	___X_____X_____

FITNESS CLASS

(or any physical activity-walk, jog, squash)

START:_____FINISH:_____

TYPE:_____

INSTRUCTOR:_____

ESTIMATE OF
CALORIES BURNED:

COMMENTS:_____

CARDIO SESSION #2

TIME:_____

ACTIVITY:_____

DURATION:_____LEVEL_____

DISTANCE:_____

CALORIES BURNED:_____

ACTIVITY PULSE RATE:_____bpm

RECOVERY PULSE RATE:_____bpm

DIFFERENCE:_____

COMMENTS:_____

TOTAL CALORIES
BURNED TODAY:

Daily Nutrition Tracking

NUTRITION	Points Goal	CAL *option*	PROT *grams*	FAT *grams*	CARB *grams*
Meal #1 – Time: H₂O____Cups(L)					
Meal #2 – Time: H₂O____Cups(L)					
Meal #3 – Time: H₂O____Cups(L)					
Meal #4 – Time: H₂O____Cups(L)					
Meal #5 – Time: H₂O____Cups(L)					
Meal #6 – Time: H₂O____Cups(L)					

Food Point Total For Today:					
Difference *(Goal Points Minus Actual Points)*					
Daily Totals: *(Add up each nutrient column. Convert each to calories. Add all and enter in "Total Calories")*			*g*	*g*	*g*

3

Conversion To Calories Multiply Total Grams of **Pro X 4** = Calories Multiply Total Grams of **Carb X 4**=Calories Multiply Total Grams of **Fat X 9** = Calories	**Total Calories**	*cal*	*cal*	*cal*
Daily Percentages: (*Divide total calories of each nutrient by the Total Number of Calories*)		__ *%*	__ *%*	__ *%*

Total Calories Consumed:_____

                    VS   *Difference*

Total Calories Burned: _____

Personal Training Log

WEIGHT TRAINING

Date:_____ Phase:_____

Start:_____ Finish:_____ Duration:_____

Day:_____ Warm Up:_____

EXERCISE	SET X REPS X WEIGHT @ TEMPO
1.	___X___X_____@__/__/__
	___X___X_____@__/__/__
	___X___X_____@__/__/__
	___X___X_____@__/__/__
	___X___X_____@__/__/__
2.	___X___X_____@__/__/__
	___X___X_____@__/__/__
	___X___X_____@__/__/__
	___X___X_____@__/__/__
	___X___X_____@__/__/__
3.	___X___X_____@__/__/__
	___X___X_____@__/__/__
	___X___X_____@__/__/__
	___X___X_____@__/__/__
	___X___X_____@__/__/__
4.	___X___X_____@__/__/__
	___X___X_____@__/__/__
	___X___X_____@__/__/__
	___X___X_____@__/__/__
	___X___X_____@__/__/__
5.	___X___X_____@__/__/__
	___X___X_____@__/__/__
	___X___X_____@__/__/__
	___X___X_____@__/__/__
	___X___X_____@__/__/__
6.	___X___X_____@__/__/__
	___X___X_____@__/__/__
	___X___X_____@__/__/__
	___X___X_____@__/__/__
	___X___X_____@__/__/__
7.	___X___X_____@__/__/__
	___X___X_____@__/__/__
	___X___X_____@__/__/__
	___X___X_____@__/__/__
	___X___X_____@__/__/__
8.	___X___X_____@__/__/__
	___X___X_____@__/__/__
	___X___X_____@__/__/__
	___X___X_____@__/__/__
	___X___X_____@__/__/__
9.	___X___X_____@__/__/__
	___X___X_____@__/__/__
	___X___X_____@__/__/__
	___X___X_____@__/__/__
	___X___X_____@__/__/__

CARDIO SESSION #1

TIME:_____

ACTIVITY:_____

DURATION:_____ LEVEL_____

DISTANCE:_____

CALORIES BURNED:_____

ACTIVITY PULSE RATE:_____bpm

RECOVERY PULSE RATE:_____bpm

DIFFERENCE:

DAILY SLEEP TRACKER

TIME TO BED:_____

TIME UP:_____

HOURS OF SLEEP:_____

COMMENTS:_____

DAILY AB TRACKER

EXERCISE	SET X REPS X WGT
1._____	___X___X_____
2._____	___X___X_____
3._____	___X___X_____
4._____	___X___X_____
5._____	___X___X_____

FITNESS CLASS

(or any physical activity-walk, jog, squash)

START:_____ FINISH:_____

TYPE:_____

INSTRUCTOR:_____

ESTIMATE OF
CALORIES BURNED:

COMMENTS:_____

CARDIO SESSION #2

TIME:_____

ACTIVITY:_____

DURATION:_____ LEVEL_____

DISTANCE:_____

CALORIES BURNED:_____

ACTIVITY PULSE RATE:_____bpm

RECOVERY PULSE RATE:_____bpm

DIFFERENCE:_____

COMMENTS:_____

TOTAL CALORIES
BURNED TODAY:

Daily Nutrition Tracking

NUTRITION	Points Goal	CAL *option*	PROT *grams*	FAT *grams*	CARB *grams*
Meal #1 – Time: H₂O____Cups(L)					
Meal #2 – Time: H₂O____Cups(L)					
Meal #3 – Time: H₂O____Cups(L)					
Meal #4 – Time: H₂O____Cups(L)					
Meal #5 – Time: H₂O____Cups(L)					
Meal #6 – Time: H₂O____Cups(L)					
Food Point Total For Today:					
Difference (Goal Points Minus Actual Points)					

Daily Totals: *(Add up each nutrient column. Convert each to calories. Add all and enter in "Total Calories")* — g g g

Conversion To Calories
Multiply Total Grams of **Pro X 4** = Calories
Multiply Total Grams of **Carb X 4** = Calories
Multiply Total Grams of **Fat X 9** = Calories

Total Calories — cal cal cal

Daily Percentages: (Divide total calories of each nutrient by the Total Number of Calories) — % % %

Total Calories Consumed: _____
VS   **Difference**
Total Calories Burned: _____

3

Personal Training Log

WEIGHT TRAINING

Date:_____ Phase:_____

Start:_____ Finish:_____ Duration:_____

Day:_____ Warm Up:_____

EXERCISE	SET X REPS X WEIGHT @ TEMPO
1.	___X___X_____@__/__/__
	___X___X_____@__/__/__
	___X___X_____@__/__/__
	___X___X_____@__/__/__
	___X___X_____@__/__/__
2.	___X___X_____@__/__/__
	___X___X_____@__/__/__
	___X___X_____@__/__/__
	___X___X_____@__/__/__
	___X___X_____@__/__/__
3.	___X___X_____@__/__/__
	___X___X_____@__/__/__
	___X___X_____@__/__/__
	___X___X_____@__/__/__
	___X___X_____@__/__/__
4.	___X___X_____@__/__/__
	___X___X_____@__/__/__
	___X___X_____@__/__/__
	___X___X_____@__/__/__
	___X___X_____@__/__/__
5.	___X___X_____@__/__/__
	___X___X_____@__/__/__
	___X___X_____@__/__/__
	___X___X_____@__/__/__
	___X___X_____@__/__/__
6.	___X___X_____@__/__/__
	___X___X_____@__/__/__
	___X___X_____@__/__/__
	___X___X_____@__/__/__
	___X___X_____@__/__/__
7.	___X___X_____@__/__/__
	___X___X_____@__/__/__
	___X___X_____@__/__/__
	___X___X_____@__/__/__
	___X___X_____@__/__/__
8.	___X___X_____@__/__/__
	___X___X_____@__/__/__
	___X___X_____@__/__/__
	___X___X_____@__/__/__
	___X___X_____@__/__/__
9.	___X___X_____@__/__/__
	___X___X_____@__/__/__
	___X___X_____@__/__/__
	___X___X_____@__/__/__
	___X___X_____@__/__/__

CARDIO SESSION #1

TIME:_____

ACTIVITY:_____

DURATION:_____ LEVEL_____

DISTANCE:_____

CALORIES BURNED:_____

ACTIVITY PULSE RATE:_____bpm

RECOVERY PULSE RATE:_____bpm

DIFFERENCE:

DAILY SLEEP TRACKER

TIME TO BED:_____

TIME UP:_____

HOURS OF SLEEP:_____

COMMENTS:_____

DAILY AB TRACKER

EXERCISE	SET X REPS X WGT
1._____	___X___X_____
2._____	___X___X_____
3._____	___X___X_____
4._____	___X___X_____
5._____	___X___X_____

FITNESS CLASS
(or any physical activity-walk, jog, squash)

START:_____ FINISH:_____

TYPE:_____

INSTRUCTOR:_____

ESTIMATE OF
CALORIES BURNED:

COMMENTS:_____

CARDIO SESSION #2

TIME:_____

ACTIVITY:_____

DURATION:_____ LEVEL_____

DISTANCE:_____

CALORIES BURNED:_____

ACTIVITY PULSE RATE:_____bpm

RECOVERY PULSE RATE:_____bpm

DIFFERENCE:_____

COMMENTS:_____

_____

TOTAL CALORIES
BURNED TODAY:

NUTRITION	Points Goal	CAL *option*	PROT *grams*	FAT *grams*	CARB *grams*
Meal #1 – Time: H$_2$O_____Cups(L)					
Meal #2 – Time: H$_2$O_____Cups(L)					
Meal #3 – Time: H$_2$O_____Cups(L)					
Meal #4 – Time: H$_2$O_____Cups(L)					
Meal #5 – Time: H$_2$O_____Cups(L)					
Meal #6 – Time: H$_2$O_____Cups(L)					

Food Point Total For Today:					
Difference *(Goal Points Minus Actual Points)*					
Daily Totals: *(Add up each nutrient column. Convert each to calories. Add all and enter in "Total Calories")*			g	g	g
Conversion To Calories Multiply Total Grams of **Pro X 4** = Calories / Multiply Total Grams of **Carb X 4**=Calories / Multiply Total Grams of **Fat X 9** = Calories	**Total Calories**		cal	cal	cal
Daily Percentages: *(Divide total calories of each nutrient by the Total Number of Calories)*			___ %	___ %	___ %

3

Total Calories Consumed:_____

                    VS   **Difference**

Total Calories Burned: _____

Personal Training Log

WEIGHT TRAINING

Date:_____ Phase:_____

Start:_____ Finish:_____ Duration:_____

Day:_____ Warm Up:_____

EXERCISE	SET X REPS X WEIGHT @ TEMPO
1.	___ X ___ X _____ @__/__/__
	___ X ___ X _____ @__/__/__
	___ X ___ X _____ @__/__/__
	___ X ___ X _____ @__/__/__
	___ X ___ X _____ @__/__/__
2.	___ X ___ X _____ @__/__/__
	___ X ___ X _____ @__/__/__
	___ X ___ X _____ @__/__/__
	___ X ___ X _____ @__/__/__
	___ X ___ X _____ @__/__/__
3.	___ X ___ X _____ @__/__/__
	___ X ___ X _____ @__/__/__
	___ X ___ X _____ @__/__/__
	___ X ___ X _____ @__/__/__
	___ X ___ X _____ @__/__/__
4.	___ X ___ X _____ @__/__/__
	___ X ___ X _____ @__/__/__
	___ X ___ X _____ @__/__/__
	___ X ___ X _____ @__/__/__
	___ X ___ X _____ @__/__/__
5.	___ X ___ X _____ @__/__/__
	___ X ___ X _____ @__/__/__
	___ X ___ X _____ @__/__/__
	___ X ___ X _____ @__/__/__
	___ X ___ X _____ @__/__/__
6.	___ X ___ X _____ @__/__/__
	___ X ___ X _____ @__/__/__
	___ X ___ X _____ @__/__/__
	___ X ___ X _____ @__/__/__
	___ X ___ X _____ @__/__/__
7.	___ X ___ X _____ @__/__/__
	___ X ___ X _____ @__/__/__
	___ X ___ X _____ @__/__/__
	___ X ___ X _____ @__/__/__
	___ X ___ X _____ @__/__/__
8.	___ X ___ X _____ @__/__/__
	___ X ___ X _____ @__/__/__
	___ X ___ X _____ @__/__/__
	___ X ___ X _____ @__/__/__
	___ X ___ X _____ @__/__/__
9.	___ X ___ X _____ @__/__/__
	___ X ___ X _____ @__/__/__
	___ X ___ X _____ @__/__/__
	___ X ___ X _____ @__/__/__
	___ X ___ X _____ @__/__/__

3

CARDIO SESSION #1

TIME:_____

ACTIVITY:_____

DURATION:_____ LEVEL_____

DISTANCE:_____

CALORIES BURNED:_____

ACTIVITY PULSE RATE:_____bpm

RECOVERY PULSE RATE:_____bpm

DIFFERENCE:

DAILY SLEEP TRACKER

TIME TO BED:_____

TIME UP:_____

HOURS OF SLEEP:_____

COMMENTS:_____

DAILY AB TRACKER

EXERCISE	SET X REPS X WGT
1._____	___ X ___ X _____
2._____	___ X ___ X _____
3._____	___ X ___ X _____
4._____	___ X ___ X _____
5._____	___ X ___ X _____

FITNESS CLASS
(or any physical activity-walk, jog, squash)

START:_____ FINISH:_____

TYPE:_____

INSTRUCTOR:_____

ESTIMATE OF
CALORIES BURNED:

COMMENTS:_____

CARDIO SESSION #2

TIME:_____

ACTIVITY:_____

DURATION:_____ LEVEL_____

DISTANCE:_____

CALORIES BURNED:_____

ACTIVITY PULSE RATE:_____bpm

RECOVERY PULSE RATE:_____bpm

DIFFERENCE:_____

COMMENTS:_____

TOTAL CALORIES
BURNED TODAY:

Daily Nutrition Tracking

NUTRITION	Points Goal	CAL *option*	PROT *grams*	FAT *grams*	CARB *grams*
Meal #1 – Time: H$_2$O____Cups(L)					
Meal #2 – Time: H$_2$O____Cups(L)					
Meal #3 – Time: H$_2$O____Cups(L)					
Meal #4 – Time: H$_2$O____Cups(L)					
Meal #5 – Time: H$_2$O____Cups(L)					
Meal #6 – Time: H$_2$O____Cups(L)					

Food Point Total For Today:					
Difference (Goal Points Minus Actual Points)					
Daily Totals: (Add up each nutrient column. Convert each to calories. Add all and enter in "Total Calories")			g	g	g
Conversion To Calories Multiply Total Grams of **Pro X 4** = Calories Multiply Total Grams of **Carb X 4**=Calories Multiply Total Grams of **Fat X 9** – Calories	***Total Calories***		cal	cal	cal
Daily Percentages: (Divide total calories of each nutrient by the Total Number of Calories)			%	%	%

Total Calories Consumed: _____
VS   ***Difference***
Total Calories Burned: _____

3

Personal Training Log

WEIGHT TRAINING

Date:_____ Phase:_____

Start:_____ Finish:_____ Duration:_____

Day:_____ Warm Up:_____

EXERCISE	SET X REPS X WEIGHT @ TEMPO
1.	___X___X___@___/___/___
	___X___X___@___/___/___
	___X___X___@___/___/___
	___X___X___@___/___/___
	___X___X___@___/___/___
2.	___X___X___@___/___/___
	___X___X___@___/___/___
	___X___X___@___/___/___
	___X___X___@___/___/___
	___X___X___@___/___/___
3.	___X___X___@___/___/___
	___X___X___@___/___/___
	___X___X___@___/___/___
	___X___X___@___/___/___
	___X___X___@___/___/___
4.	___X___X___@___/___/___
	___X___X___@___/___/___
	___X___X___@___/___/___
	___X___X___@___/___/___
	___X___X___@___/___/___
5.	___X___X___@___/___/___
	___X___X___@___/___/___
	___X___X___@___/___/___
	___X___X___@___/___/___
	___X___X___@___/___/___
6.	___X___X___@___/___/___
	___X___X___@___/___/___
	___X___X___@___/___/___
	___X___X___@___/___/___
	___X___X___@___/___/___
7.	___X___X___@___/___/___
	___X___X___@___/___/___
	___X___X___@___/___/___
	___X___X___@___/___/___
	___X___X___@___/___/___
8.	___X___X___@___/___/___
	___X___X___@___/___/___
	___X___X___@___/___/___
	___X___X___@___/___/___
	___X___X___@___/___/___
9.	___X___X___@___/___/___
	___X___X___@___/___/___
	___X___X___@___/___/___
	___X___X___@___/___/___
	___X___X___@___/___/___

CARDIO SESSION #1

TIME:_____

ACTIVITY:_____

DURATION:_____ LEVEL_____

DISTANCE:_____

CALORIES BURNED:_____

ACTIVITY PULSE RATE:_____bpm

RECOVERY PULSE RATE:_____bpm

DIFFERENCE:

DAILY SLEEP TRACKER

TIME TO BED:_____

TIME UP:_____

HOURS OF SLEEP:_____

COMMENTS:_____

DAILY AB TRACKER

EXERCISE	SET X REPS X WGT
1._____	___X___X___
2._____	___X___X___
3._____	___X___X___
4._____	___X___X___
5._____	___X___X___

FITNESS CLASS

(or any physical activity-walk, jog, squash)

START:_____ FINISH:_____

TYPE:_____

INSTRUCTOR:_____

ESTIMATE OF
CALORIES BURNED: [ ]

COMMENTS:_____

CARDIO SESSION #2

TIME:_____

ACTIVITY:_____

DURATION:_____ LEVEL_____

DISTANCE:_____

CALORIES BURNED:_____

ACTIVITY PULSE RATE:_____bpm

RECOVERY PULSE RATE:_____bpm

DIFFERENCE:_____

COMMENTS:_____

TOTAL CALORIES
BURNED TODAY: [ ]

Daily Nutrition Tracking

NUTRITION	Points Goal	CAL *option*	PROT *grams*	FAT *grams*	CARB *grams*
Meal #1 – Time: H₂O____Cups(L)					
Meal #2 – Time: H₂O____Cups(L)					
Meal #3 – Time: H₂O____Cups(L)					
Meal #4 – Time: H₂O____Cups(L)					
Meal #5 – Time: H₂O____Cups(L)					
Meal #6 – Time: H₂O____Cups(L)					

Food Point Total For Today:

Difference (Goal Points Minus Actual Points)

3

Daily Totals: *(Add up each nutrient column. Convert each to calories. Add all and enter in "Total Calories")* — g | g | g

Conversion To Calories | **Total Calories**
Multiply Total Grams of **Pro X 4** = Calories
Multiply Total Grams of **Carb X 4** = Calories
Multiply Total Grams of **Fat X 9** = Calories — cal | cal | cal

Daily Percentages: (Divide total calories of each nutrient by the Total Number of Calories) — % | % | %

Total Calories Consumed:_____
VS **Difference**
Total Calories Burned: _____

Personal Training Log

WEIGHT TRAINING

Date:_____ Phase:_____

Start:_____ Finish:_____ Duration:_____

Day:_____ Warm Up:_____

EXERCISE	SET X REPS X WEIGHT @ TEMPO
1.	___X_____X_____ @___/___/___
	___X_____X_____ @___/___/___
	___X_____X_____ @___/___/___
	___X_____X_____ @___/___/___
	___X_____X_____ @___/___/___
2.	___X_____X_____ @___/___/___
	___X_____X_____ @___/___/___
	___X_____X_____ @___/___/___
	___X_____X_____ @___/___/___
	___X_____X_____ @___/___/___
3.	___X_____X_____ @___/___/___
	___X_____X_____ @___/___/___
	___X_____X_____ @___/___/___
	___X_____X_____ @___/___/___
	___X_____X_____ @___/___/___
4.	___X_____X_____ @___/___/___
	___X_____X_____ @___/___/___
	___X_____X_____ @___/___/___
	___X_____X_____ @___/___/___
	___X_____X_____ @___/___/___
5.	___X_____X_____ @___/___/___
	___X_____X_____ @___/___/___
	___X_____X_____ @___/___/___
	___X_____X_____ @___/___/___
	___X_____X_____ @___/___/___
6.	___X_____X_____ @___/___/___
	___X_____X_____ @___/___/___
	___X_____X_____ @___/___/___
	___X_____X_____ @___/___/___
	___X_____X_____ @___/___/___
7.	___X_____X_____ @___/___/___
	___X_____X_____ @___/___/___
	___X_____X_____ @___/___/___
	___X_____X_____ @___/___/___
	___X_____X_____ @___/___/___
8.	___X_____X_____ @___/___/___
	___X_____X_____ @___/___/___
	___X_____X_____ @___/___/___
	___X_____X_____ @___/___/___
	___X_____X_____ @___/___/___
9.	___X_____X_____ @___/___/___
	___X_____X_____ @___/___/___
	___X_____X_____ @___/___/___
	___X_____X_____ @___/___/___
	___X_____X_____ @___/___/___

CARDIO SESSION #1

TIME:_____

ACTIVITY:_____

DURATION:_____ LEVEL_____

DISTANCE:_____

CALORIES BURNED:_____

ACTIVITY PULSE RATE:_____bpm

RECOVERY PULSE RATE:_____bpm

DIFFERENCE:

DAILY SLEEP TRACKER

TIME TO BED:_____

TIME UP:_____

HOURS OF SLEEP:_____

COMMENTS:_____

DAILY AB TRACKER

EXERCISE	SET X REPS X WGT
1._____	___X_____X_____
2._____	___X_____X_____
3._____	___X_____X_____
4._____	___X_____X_____
5._____	___X_____X_____

FITNESS CLASS
(or any physical activity-walk, jog, squash)

START:_____ FINISH:_____

TYPE:_____

INSTRUCTOR:_____

ESTIMATE OF
CALORIES BURNED:

COMMENTS:_____

CARDIO SESSION #2

TIME:_____

ACTIVITY:_____

DURATION:_____ LEVEL_____

DISTANCE:_____

CALORIES BURNED:_____

ACTIVITY PULSE RATE:_____bpm

RECOVERY PULSE RATE:_____bpm

DIFFERENCE:_____

COMMENTS:_____

TOTAL CALORIES
BURNED TODAY:

3

NUTRITION	Points Goal	CAL *option*	PROT *grams*	FAT *grams*	CARB *grams*
Meal #1 – Time: H₂O_____Cups(L)					
Meal #2 – Time: H₂O_____Cups(L)					
Meal #3 – Time: H₂O_____Cups(L)					
Meal #4 – Time: H₂O_____Cups(L)					
Meal #5 – Time: H₂O_____Cups(L)					
Meal #6 – Time: H₂O_____Cups(L)					

Food Point Total For Today:					
Difference *(Goal Points Minus Actual Points)*					

3

Daily Totals: *(Add up each nutrient column. Convert each to calories. Add all and enter in "Total Calories")*			g	g	g
Conversion To Calories *Multiply Total Grams of **Pro X 4** = Calories* *Multiply Total Grams of **Carb X 4**=Calories* *Multiply Total Grams of **Fat X 9** = Calories*	***Total*** ***Calories***		cal	cal	cal
Daily Percentages: *(Divide total calories of each nutrient by the Total Number of Calories)*			__ %	__ %	__ %

Total Calories Consumed:_____
            VS   ***Difference***
Total Calories Burned: _____

Personal Training Log

WEIGHT TRAINING

Date:_____ Phase:_____

Start:_____ Finish:_____ Duration:_____

Day:_____ Warm Up:_____

EXERCISE	SET X REPS X WEIGHT @ TEMPO
1.	___X___X_____@__/__/__
	___X___X_____@__/__/__
	___X___X_____@__/__/__
	___X___X_____@__/__/__
	___X___X_____@__/__/__
2.	___X___X_____@__/__/__
	___X___X_____@__/__/__
	___X___X_____@__/__/__
	___X___X_____@__/__/__
	___X___X_____@__/__/__
3.	___X___X_____@__/__/__
	___X___X_____@__/__/__
	___X___X_____@__/__/__
	___X___X_____@__/__/__
	___X___X_____@__/__/__
4.	___X___X_____@__/__/__
	___X___X_____@__/__/__
	___X___X_____@__/__/__
	___X___X_____@__/__/__
	___X___X_____@__/__/__
5.	___X___X_____@__/__/__
	___X___X_____@__/__/__
	___X___X_____@__/__/__
	___X___X_____@__/__/__
	___X___X_____@__/__/__
6.	___X___X_____@__/__/__
	___X___X_____@__/__/__
	___X___X_____@__/__/__
	___X___X_____@__/__/__
	___X___X_____@__/__/__
7.	___X___X_____@__/__/__
	___X___X_____@__/__/__
	___X___X_____@__/__/__
	___X___X_____@__/__/__
8.	___X___X_____@__/__/__
	___X___X_____@__/__/__
	___X___X_____@__/__/__
	___X___X_____@__/__/__
	___X___X_____@__/__/__
9.	___X___X_____@__/__/__
	___X___X_____@__/__/__
	___X___X_____@__/__/__
	___X___X_____@__/__/__
	___X___X_____@__/__/__

CARDIO SESSION #1

TIME:_____

ACTIVITY:_____

DURATION:_____ LEVEL_____

DISTANCE:_____

CALORIES BURNED:_____

ACTIVITY PULSE RATE:_____bpm

RECOVERY PULSE RATE:_____bpm

DIFFERENCE:

DAILY SLEEP TRACKER

TIME TO BED:_____

TIME UP:_____

HOURS OF SLEEP:_____

COMMENTS:_____

DAILY AB TRACKER

EXERCISE	SET X REPS X WGT
1._____	___X____X_____
2._____	___X____X_____
3._____	___X____X_____
4._____	___X____X_____
5._____	___X____X_____

FITNESS CLASS

(or any physical activity-walk, jog, squash)

START:_____ FINISH:_____

TYPE:_____

INSTRUCTOR:_____

ESTIMATE OF
CALORIES BURNED: [____]

COMMENTS:_____

CARDIO SESSION #2

TIME:_____

ACTIVITY:_____

DURATION:_____ LEVEL_____

DISTANCE:

CALORIES BURNED:_____

ACTIVITY PULSE RATE:_____bpm

RECOVERY PULSE RATE:_____bpm

DIFFERENCE:_____

COMMENTS:_____

TOTAL CALORIES
BURNED TODAY: [____]

NUTRITION	Points Goal	CAL *option*	PROT *grams*	FAT *grams*	CARB *grams*
Meal #1 – Time: H₂O_____Cups(L)					
Meal #2 – Time: H₂O_____Cups(L)					
Meal #3 – Time: H₂O_____Cups(L)					
Meal #4 – Time: H₂O_____Cups(L)					
Meal #5 – Time: H₂O_____Cups(L)					
Meal #6 – Time: H₂O_____Cups(L)					

Food Point Total For Today:		
Difference (Goal Points Minus Actual Points)		

3

Daily Totals: (Add up each nutrient column. Convert each to calories. Add all and enter in "Total Calories")   *g*   *g*   *g*

Conversion To Calories
Multiply Total Grams of **Pro X 4** = Calories
Multiply Total Grams of **Carb X 4**=Calories
Multiply Total Grams of **Fat X 9** = Calories

Total Calories

    cal   *cal*   *cal*

Daily Percentages: (Divide total calories of each nutrient by the Total Number of Calories)   *%*   *%*   *%*

Total Calories Consumed:_____
      VS   **Difference**
Total Calories Burned: _____

Personal Training Log

WEIGHT TRAINING

Date:_____ Phase:_____

Start:_____ Finish:_____ Duration:_____

Day:_____ Warm Up:_____

EXERCISE	SET X REPS X WEIGHT @ TEMPO
1.	___X___X_____@__/__/__
	___X___X_____@__/__/__
	___X___X_____@__/__/__
	___X___X_____@__/__/__
	___X___X_____@__/__/__
2.	___X___X_____@__/__/__
	___X___X_____@__/__/__
	___X___X_____@__/__/__
	___X___X_____@__/__/__
	___X___X_____@__/__/__
3.	___X___X_____@__/__/__
	___X___X_____@__/__/__
	___X___X_____@__/__/__
	___X___X_____@__/__/__
	___X___X_____@__/__/__
4.	___X___X_____@__/__/__
	___X___X_____@__/__/__
	___X___X_____@__/__/__
	___X___X_____@__/__/__
	___X___X_____@__/__/__
5.	___X___X_____@__/__/__
	___X___X_____@__/__/__
	___X___X_____@__/__/__
	___X___X_____@__/__/__
	___X___X_____@__/__/__
6.	___X___X_____@__/__/__
	___X___X_____@__/__/__
	___X___X_____@__/__/__
	___X___X_____@__/__/__
	___X___X_____@__/__/__
7.	___X___X_____@__/__/__
	___X___X_____@__/__/__
	___X___X_____@__/__/__
	___X___X_____@__/__/__
	___X___X_____@__/__/__
8.	___X___X_____@__/__/__
	___X___X_____@__/__/__
	___X___X_____@__/__/__
	___X___X_____@__/__/__
	___A___A_____@__/__/__
9.	___X___X_____@__/__/__
	___X___X_____@__/__/__
	___X___X_____@__/__/__
	___X___X_____@__/__/__
	___X___X_____@__/__/__

CARDIO SESSION #1

TIME:_____

ACTIVITY:_____

DURATION:_____ LEVEL_____

DISTANCE:_____

CALORIES BURNED:_____

ACTIVITY PULSE RATE:_____bpm

RECOVERY PULSE RATE:_____bpm

DIFFERENCE:

DAILY SLEEP TRACKER

TIME TO BED:_____

TIME UP:_____

HOURS OF SLEEP:_____

COMMENTS:_____

DAILY AB TRACKER

EXERCISE	SET X REPS X WGT
1._____	___X___X___
2._____	___X___X___
3._____	___X___X___
4._____	___X___X___
5._____	___X___X___

FITNESS CLASS

(or any physical activity-walk, jog, squash)

START:_____ FINISH:_____

TYPE:_____

INSTRUCTOR:_____

ESTIMATE OF
CALORIES BURNED: [____]

COMMENTS:_____

CARDIO SESSION #2

TIME:_____

ACTIVITY:_____

DURATION:_____ LEVEL_____

DISTANCE:_____

CALORIES BURNED:_____

ACTIVITY PULSE RATE:_____bpm

RECOVERY PULSE RATE:_____bpm

DIFFERENCE:_____

COMMENTS:_____

TOTAL CALORIES
BURNED TODAY: [____]

Daily Nutrition Tracking

NUTRITION	Points Goal	CAL *option*	PROT *grams*	FAT *grams*	CARB *grams*
Meal #1 – Time: H₂O____Cups(L)					
Meal #2 – Time: H₂O____Cups(L)					
Meal #3 – Time: H₂O____Cups(L)					
Meal #4 – Time: H₂O____Cups(L)					
Meal #5 – Time: H₂O____Cups(L)					
Meal #6 – Time: H₂O____Cups(L)					

Food Point Total For Today:

Difference (Goal Points Minus Actual Points)

Daily Totals: *(Add up each nutrient column. Convert each to calories. Add all and enter in "Total Calories")* — g | g | g

Conversion To Calories — Multiply Total Grams of **Pro X 4** = Calories; Multiply Total Grams of **Carb X 4** = Calories; Multiply Total Grams of **Fat X 9** = Calories — **Total Calories** — cal | cal | cal

Daily Percentages: *(Divide total calories of each nutrient by the Total Number of Calories)* — % | % | %

Total Calories Consumed:_____
VS   **Difference**
Total Calories Burned:_____

3

Personal Training Log

<table>
<tr><td colspan="2" align="center"><u>WEIGHT TRAINING</u></td><td colspan="2" align="center">CARDIO SESSION #1</td></tr>
</table>

WEIGHT TRAINING

Date:_____ Phase:_____

Start:_____ Finish:_____ Duration:_____

Day:_____ Warm Up:_____

EXERCISE	SET X REPS X WEIGHT @ TEMPO
1.	___ X ___ X _____ @ __/__/__
	___ X ___ X _____ @ __/__/__
	___ X ___ X _____ @ __/__/__
	___ X ___ X _____ @ __/__/__
	___ X ___ X _____ @ __/__/__
2.	___ X ___ X _____ @ __/__/__
	___ X ___ X _____ @ __/__/__
	___ X ___ X _____ @ __/__/__
	___ X ___ X _____ @ __/__/__
	___ X ___ X _____ @ __/__/__
3.	___ X ___ X _____ @ __/__/__
	___ X ___ X _____ @ __/__/__
	___ X ___ X _____ @ __/__/__
	___ X ___ X _____ @ __/__/__
	___ X ___ X _____ @ __/__/__
4.	___ X ___ X _____ @ __/__/__
	___ X ___ X _____ @ __/__/__
	___ X ___ X _____ @ __/__/__
	___ X ___ X _____ @ __/__/__
	___ X ___ X _____ @ __/__/__
5.	___ X ___ X _____ @ __/__/__
	___ X ___ X _____ @ __/__/__
	___ X ___ X _____ @ __/__/__
	___ X ___ X _____ @ __/__/__
	___ X ___ X _____ @ __/__/__
6.	___ X ___ X _____ @ __/__/__
	___ X ___ X _____ @ __/__/__
	___ X ___ X _____ @ __/__/__
	___ X ___ X _____ @ __/__/__
	___ X ___ X _____ @ __/__/__
7.	___ X ___ X _____ @ __/__/__
	___ X ___ X _____ @ __/__/__
	___ X ___ X _____ @ __/__/__
	___ X ___ X _____ @ __/__/__
	___ X ___ X _____ @ __/__/__
8.	___ X ___ X _____ @ __/__/__
	___ X ___ X _____ @ __/__/__
	___ X ___ X _____ @ __/__/__
	___ X ___ X _____ @ __/__/__
	___ X ___ X _____ @ __/__/__
9.	___ X ___ X _____ @ __/__/__
	___ X ___ X _____ @ __/__/__
	___ X ___ X _____ @ __/__/__
	___ X ___ X _____ @ __/__/__
	___ X ___ X _____ @ __/__/__

CARDIO SESSION #1

TIME:_____

ACTIVITY:_____

DURATION:_____ LEVEL_____

DISTANCE:_____

CALORIES BURNED:_____

ACTIVITY PULSE RATE:_____bpm

RECOVERY PULSE RATE:_____bpm

DIFFERENCE:

DAILY SLEEP TRACKER

TIME TO BED:_____

TIME UP:_____

HOURS OF SLEEP:_____

COMMENTS:_____

DAILY AB TRACKER

EXERCISE	SET X REPS X WGT
1._____	___ X ___ X ___
2._____	___ X ___ X ___
3._____	___ X ___ X ___
4._____	___ X ___ X ___
5._____	___ X ___ X ___

FITNESS CLASS

(or any physical activity-walk, jog, squash)

START:_____ FINISH:_____

TYPE:_____

INSTRUCTOR:_____

ESTIMATE OF
CALORIES BURNED: [_____]

COMMENTS:_____

CARDIO SESSION #2

TIME:_____

ACTIVITY:_____

DURATION:_____ LEVEL_____

DISTANCE:_____

CALORIES BURNED:_____

ACTIVITY PULSE RATE:_____bpm

RECOVERY PULSE RATE:_____bpm

DIFFERENCE:_____

COMMENTS:_____

_____

TOTAL CALORIES
BURNED TODAY: [_____]

Daily Nutrition Tracking

NUTRITION	Points Goal	CAL *option*	PROT *grams*	FAT *grams*	CARB *grams*
Meal #1 – Time: H₂O____Cups(L)					
Meal #2 – Time: H₂O____Cups(L)					
Meal #3 – Time: H₂O____Cups(L)					
Meal #4 – Time: H₂O____Cups(L)					
Meal #5 – Time: H₂O____Cups(L)					
Meal #6 – Time: H₂O____Cups(L)					

Food Point Total For Today:					
Difference *(Goal Points Minus Actual Points)*					
Daily Totals:*(Add up each nutrient column. Convert each to calories. Add all and enter in "Total Calories")*			g	g	g

Conversion To Calories Multiply Total Grams of **Pro X 4** = Calories Multiply Total Grams of **Carb X 4**=Calories Multiply Total Grams of **Fat X 9** = Calories	***Total Calories***	cal	cal	cal

Daily Percentages: *(Divide total calories of each nutrient by the Total Number of Calories)*	%	%	%

***Total Calories Consumed:*_____**
          VS   ***Difference***
***Total Calories Burned:* _____**

3

Personal Training Log

WEIGHT TRAINING

Date:_____ Phase:_____

Start:_____ Finish:_____ Duration:_____

Day:_____ Warm Up:_____

EXERCISE	SET X REPS X WEIGHT @ TEMPO
1.	___X___X _____@__/__/__
	___X___X _____@__/__/__
	___X___X _____@__/__/__
	___X___X _____@__/__/__
	___X___X _____@__/__/__
2.	___X___X _____@__/__/__
	___X___X _____@__/__/__
	___X___X _____@__/__/__
	___X___X _____@__/__/__
	___X___X _____@__/__/__
3.	___X___X _____@__/__/__
	___X___X _____@__/__/__
	___X___X _____@__/__/__
	___X___X _____@__/__/__
	___X___X _____@__/__/__
4.	___X___X _____@__/__/__
	___X___X _____@__/__/__
	___X___X _____@__/__/__
	___X___X _____@__/__/__
	___X___X _____@__/__/__
5.	___X___X _____@__/__/__
	___X___X _____@__/__/__
	___X___X _____@__/__/__
	___X___X _____@__/__/__
	___X___X _____@__/__/__
6.	___X___X _____@__/__/__
	___X___X _____@__/__/__
	___X___X _____@__/__/__
	___X___X _____@__/__/__
	___X___X _____@__/__/__
7.	___X___X _____@__/__/__
	___X___X _____@__/__/__
	___X___X _____@__/__/__
	___X___X _____@__/__/__
	___X___X _____@__/__/__
8.	___X___X _____@__/__/__
	___X___X _____@__/__/__
	___X___X _____@__/__/__
	___X___X _____@__/__/__
	___X___X _____@__/__/__
9.	___X___X _____@__/__/__
	___X___X _____@__/__/__
	___X___X _____@__/__/__
	___X___X _____@__/__/__
	___X___X _____@__/__/__

CARDIO SESSION #1

TIME:_____

ACTIVITY:_____

DURATION:_____ LEVEL_____

DISTANCE:_____

CALORIES BURNED:_____

ACTIVITY PULSE RATE:_____bpm

RECOVERY PULSE RATE:_____bpm

DIFFERENCE:

DAILY SLEEP TRACKER

TIME TO BED:_____

TIME UP:_____

HOURS OF SLEEP:_____

COMMENTS:_____

DAILY AB TRACKER

EXERCISE	SET X REPS X WGT
1._____	___X___X___
2._____	___X___X___
3._____	___X___X___
4._____	___X___X___
5._____	___X___X___

FITNESS CLASS

(or any physical activity-walk, jog, squash)

START:_____ FINISH:_____

TYPE:_____

INSTRUCTOR:_____

ESTIMATE OF
CALORIES BURNED:

COMMENTS:_____

CARDIO SESSION #2

TIME:_____

ACTIVITY:_____

DURATION:_____ LEVEL_____

DISTANCE:_____

CALORIES BURNED:_____

ACTIVITY PULSE RATE:_____bpm

RECOVERY PULSE RATE:_____bpm

DIFFERENCE:_____

COMMENTS:_____

TOTAL CALORIES
BURNED TODAY:

Daily Nutrition Tracking

NUTRITION	Points Goal	CAL *option*	PROT *grams*	FAT *grams*	CARB *grams*
Meal #1 – Time: H₂O_____Cups(L)					
Meal #2 – Time: H₂O_____Cups(L)					
Meal #3 – Time: H₂O_____Cups(L)					
Meal #4 – Time: H₂O_____Cups(L)					
Meal #5 – Time: H₂O_____Cups(L)					
Meal #6 – Time: H₂O_____Cups(L)					
Food Point Total For Today:					
Difference (Goal Points Minus Actual Points)					

3

Daily Totals: *(Add up each nutrient column. Convert each to calories. Add all and enter in "Total Calories")* — g | g | g

Conversion To Calories *Multiply Total Grams of **Pro X 4** = Calories* *Multiply Total Grams of **Carb X 4**=Calories* *Multiply Total Grams of **Fat X 9** = Calories*	***Total Calories***	cal	cal	cal

Daily Percentages: *(Divide total calories of each nutrient by the Total Number of Calories)* — % | % | %

Total Calories Consumed:_____
      VS   ***Difference***   [ ]
Total Calories Burned:_____

Personal Training Log

WEIGHT TRAINING

Date:_____ Phase:_____

Start:_____ Finish:_____ Duration:_____

Day:_____ Warm Up:_____

EXERCISE	SET X REPS X WEIGHT @ TEMPO
1.	___X___X_____@___/___/___
	___X___X_____@___/___/___
	___X___X_____@___/___/___
	___X___X_____@___/___/___
	___X___X_____@___/___/___
2.	___X___X_____@___/___/___
	___X___X_____@___/___/___
	___X___X_____@___/___/___
	___X___X_____@___/___/___
	___X___X_____@___/___/___
3.	___X___X_____@___/___/___
	___X___X_____@___/___/___
	___X___X_____@___/___/___
	___X___X_____@___/___/___
	___X___X_____@___/___/___
4.	___X___X_____@___/___/___
	___X___X_____@___/___/___
	___X___X_____@___/___/___
	___X___X_____@___/___/___
	___X___X_____@___/___/___
5.	___X___X_____@___/___/___
	___X___X_____@___/___/___
	___X___X_____@___/___/___
	___X___X_____@___/___/___
	___X___X_____@___/___/___
6.	___X___X_____@___/___/___
	___X___X_____@___/___/___
	___X___X_____@___/___/___
	___X___X_____@___/___/___
	___X___X_____@___/___/___
7.	___X___X_____@___/___/___
	___X___X_____@___/___/___
	___X___X_____@___/___/___
	___X___X_____@___/___/___
	___X___X_____@___/___/___
8.	___X___X_____@___/___/___
	___X___X_____@___/___/___
	___X___X_____@___/___/___
	___X___X_____@___/___/___
	___X___X_____@___/___/___
9.	___X___X_____@___/___/___
	___X___X_____@___/___/___
	___X___X_____@___/___/___
	___X___X_____@___/___/___
	___X___X_____@___/___/___

CARDIO SESSION #1

TIME:_____

ACTIVITY:_____

DURATION:_____ LEVEL_____

DISTANCE:_____

CALORIES BURNED:_____

ACTIVITY PULSE RATE:_____bpm

RECOVERY PULSE RATE:_____bpm

DIFFERENCE:

DAILY SLEEP TRACKER

TIME TO BED:_____

TIME UP:_____

HOURS OF SLEEP:_____

COMMENTS:_____

DAILY AB TRACKER

EXERCISE	SET X REPS X WGT
1._____	___X_____X_____
2._____	___X_____X_____
3._____	___X_____X_____
4._____	___X_____X_____
5._____	___X_____X_____

FITNESS CLASS
(or any physical activity-walk, jog, squash)

START:_____ FINISH:_____

TYPE:_____

INSTRUCTOR:_____

ESTIMATE OF
CALORIES BURNED:

COMMENTS:_____

CARDIO SESSION #2

TIME:_____

ACTIVITY:_____

DURATION:_____ LEVEL_____

DISTANCE:_____

CALORIES BURNED:_____

ACTIVITY PULSE RATE:_____bpm

RECOVERY PULSE RATE:_____bpm

DIFFERENCE:_____

COMMENTS:_____

TOTAL CALORIES
BURNED TODAY:

<u>**NUTRITION**</u>	Points Goal	CAL *option*	PROT *grams*	FAT *grams*	CARB *grams*
Meal #1 – Time: H₂O_____Cups(L)					
Meal #2 – Time: H₂O_____Cups(L)					
Meal #3 – Time: H₂O_____Cups(L)					
Meal #4 – Time: H₂O_____Cups(L)					
Meal #5 – Time: H₂O_____Cups(L)					
Meal #6 – Time: H₂O_____Cups(L)					

Food Point Total For Today:					
Difference *(Goal Points Minus Actual Points)*					
Daily Totals: *(Add up each nutrient column. Convert each to calories. Add all and enter in "Total Calories")*			g	g	g
Conversion To Calories *Multiply Total Grams of **Pro X 4** = Calories* *Multiply Total Grams of **Carb X 4**=Calories* *Multiply Total Grams of **Fat X 9** = Calories*	***Total Calories***		cal	cal	cal
Daily Percentages: *(Divide total calories of each nutrient by the Total Number of Calories)*			___ %	___ %	___ %

***Total Calories Consumed:*_____**

                    VS   ***Difference***

***Total Calories Burned:* _____**

3

Personal Training Log

<table>
<tr><td colspan="3">

WEIGHT TRAINING

Date:_____ Phase:_____

Start:_____ Finish:_____ Duration:_____

Day:_____ Warm Up:_____

</td><td>

CARDIO SESSION #1

TIME:_____

ACTIVITY:_____

DURATION:_____ LEVEL_____

DISTANCE:_____

CALORIES BURNED:_____

ACTIVITY PULSE RATE:_____bpm

RECOVERY PULSE RATE:_____bpm

DIFFERENCE:

</td></tr>
</table>

EXERCISE	SET X REPS X WEIGHT @ TEMPO
1.	___X___X _____ @__/__/__
	___X___X _____ @__/__/__
	___X___X _____ @__/__/__
	___X___X _____ @__/__/__
	___X___X _____ @__/__/__

DAILY SLEEP TRACKER

TIME TO BED:_____

TIME UP:_____

HOURS OF SLEEP:_____

COMMENTS:_____

2.	___X___X _____ @__/__/__
	___X___X _____ @__/__/__
	___X___X _____ @__/__/__
	___X___X _____ @__/__/__
	___X___X _____ @__/__/__

3.	___X___X _____ @__/__/__
	___X___X _____ @__/__/__
	___X___X _____ @__/__/__
	___X___X _____ @__/__/__
	___X___X _____ @__/__/__

DAILY AB TRACKER

EXERCISE	SET X REPS X WGT
1._____	___X____X___
2._____	___X____X___
3._____	___X____X___
4._____	___X____X___
5._____	___X____X___

4.	___X___X _____ @__/__/__
	___X___X _____ @__/__/__
	___X___X _____ @__/__/__
	___X___X _____ @__/__/__
	___X___X _____ @__/__/__

5.	___X___X _____ @__/__/__
	___X___X _____ @__/__/__
	___X___X _____ @__/__/__
	___X___X _____ @__/__/__
	___X___X _____ @__/__/__

FITNESS CLASS

(or any physical activity-walk, jog, squash)

START:_____ FINISH:_____

TYPE:_____

INSTRUCTOR:_____

ESTIMATE OF
CALORIES BURNED: [   ]

6.	___X___X _____ @__/__/__
	___X___X _____ @__/__/__
	___X___X _____ @__/__/__
	___X___X _____ @__/__/__
	___X___X _____ @__/__/__

COMMENTS:_____

7.	___X___X _____ @__/__/__
	___X___X _____ @__/__/__
	___X___X _____ @__/__/__
	___X___X _____ @__/__/__
	___X___X _____ @__/__/__

CARDIO SESSION #2

TIME:_____

ACTIVITY:_____

DURATION:_____ LEVEL_____

DISTANCE:_____

8.	___X___X _____ @__/__/__
	___X___X _____ @__/__/__
	___X___X _____ @__/__/__
	___X___X _____ @__/__/__
	___X___X _____ @__/__/__

CALORIES BURNED:_____

ACTIVITY PULSE RATE:_____bpm

RECOVERY PULSE RATE:_____bpm

DIFFERENCE:_____

9.	___X___X _____ @ / /
	___X___X _____ @__/__/__
	___X___X _____ @__/__/__
	___X___X _____ @__/__/__
	___X___X _____ @__/__/__

COMMENTS:_____

_____

TOTAL CALORIES
BURNED TODAY: [   ]

3

Daily Nutrition Tracking

NUTRITION	Points Goal	CAL *option*	PROT *grams*	FAT *grams*	CARB *grams*
Meal #1 – Time: H₂O_____Cups(L)					
Meal #2 – Time: H₂O_____Cups(L)					
Meal #3 – Time: H₂O_____Cups(L)					
Meal #4 – Time: H₂O_____Cups(L)					
Meal #5 – Time: H₂O_____Cups(L)					
Meal #6 – Time: H₂O_____Cups(L)					
Food Point Total For Today:					
Difference (Goal Points Minus Actual Points)					

3

Daily Totals: (Add up each nutrient column. Convert each to calories. Add all and enter in "Total Calories")	**g**	**g**	**g**

Conversion To Calories Multiply Total Grams of ***Pro X 4*** = Calories Multiply Total Grams of ***Carb X 4***=Calories Multiply Total Grams of ***Fat X 9*** = Calories	***Total Calories***	**cal**	**cal**	**cal**

Daily Percentages: (Divide total calories of each nutrient by the Total Number of Calories)	___ %	___ %	___ %

Total Calories Consumed:_____

VS   ***Difference***

Total Calories Burned: _____

Personal Training Log

WEIGHT TRAINING

Date:_____ Phase:_____

Start:_____ Finish:_____ Duration:_____

Day:_____ Warm Up:_____

EXERCISE	SET X REPS X WEIGHT @ TEMPO
1.	___X_____X_____@__/__/__
	___X_____X_____@__/__/__
	___X_____X_____@__/__/__
	___X_____X_____@__/__/__
	___X_____X_____@__/__/__
2.	___X_____X_____@__/__/__
	___X_____X_____@__/__/__
	___X_____X_____@__/__/__
	___X_____X_____@__/__/__
	___X_____X_____@__/__/__
3.	___X_____X_____@__/__/__
	___X_____X_____@__/__/__
	___X_____X_____@__/__/__
	___X_____X_____@__/__/__
	___X_____X_____@__/__/__
4.	___X_____X_____@__/__/__
	___X_____X_____@__/__/__
	___X_____X_____@__/__/__
	___X_____X_____@__/__/__
	___X_____X_____@__/__/__
5.	___X_____X_____@__/__/__
	___X_____X_____@__/__/__
	___X_____X_____@__/__/__
	___X_____X_____@__/__/__
	___X_____X_____@__/__/__
6.	___X_____X_____@__/__/__
	___X_____X_____@__/__/__
	___X_____X_____@__/__/__
	___X_____X_____@__/__/__
	___X_____X_____@__/__/__
7.	___X_____X_____@__/__/__
	___X_____X_____@__/__/__
	___X_____X_____@__/__/__
	___X_____X_____@__/__/__
	___X_____X_____@__/__/__
8.	___X_____X_____@__/__/__
	___X_____X_____@__/__/__
	___X_____X_____@__/__/__
	___X_____X_____@__/__/__
	___X_____X_____@__/__/__
9.	___X_____X_____@__/__/__
	___X_____X_____@__/__/__
	___X_____X_____@__/__/__
	___X_____X_____@__/__/__
	___X_____X_____@__/__/__

3

CARDIO SESSION #1

TIME:_____

ACTIVITY:_____

DURATION:_____ LEVEL_____

DISTANCE:_____

CALORIES BURNED:_____

ACTIVITY PULSE RATE:_____ bpm

RECOVERY PULSE RATE:_____ bpm

DIFFERENCE:

DAILY SLEEP TRACKER

TIME TO BED:_____

TIME UP:_____

HOURS OF SLEEP:_____

COMMENTS:_____

DAILY AB TRACKER

EXERCISE	SET X REPS X WGT
1._____	___X_____X_____
2._____	___X_____X_____
3._____	___X_____X_____
4._____	___X_____X_____
5._____	___X_____X_____

FITNESS CLASS
(or any physical activity-walk, jog, squash)

START:_____ FINISH:_____

TYPE:_____

INSTRUCTOR:_____

ESTIMATE OF
CALORIES BURNED:

COMMENTS:_____

CARDIO SESSION #2

TIME:_____

ACTIVITY:_____

DURATION:_____ LEVEL_____

DISTANCE:_____

CALORIES BURNED:_____

ACTIVITY PULSE RATE:_____ bpm

RECOVERY PULSE RATE:_____ bpm

DIFFERENCE:_____

COMMENTS:_____

TOTAL CALORIES
BURNED TODAY:

NUTRITION	Points Goal	CAL *option*	PROT *grams*	FAT *grams*	CARB *grams*
Meal #1 – Time:　　　H₂O____Cups(L)					
Meal #2 – Time:　　　H₂O____Cups(L)					
Meal #3 – Time:　　　H₂O____Cups(L)					
Meal #4 – Time:　　　H₂O____Cups(L)					
Meal #5 – Time:　　　H₂O____Cups(L)					
Meal #6 – Time:　　　H₂O____Cups(L)					

Food Point Total For Today:		
Difference (Goal Points Minus Actual Points)		

3

Daily Totals: *(Add up each nutrient column. Convert each to calories. Add all and enter in "Total Calories")*　　g　g　g

Conversion To Calories
*Multiply Total Grams of **Pro X 4** = Calories*
*Multiply Total Grams of **Carb X 4**=Calories*
*Multiply Total Grams of **Fat X 9** = Calories*
Total Calories　　cal　cal　cal

Daily Percentages: (*Divide total calories of each nutrient by the Total Number of Calories*)　__%　__%　__%

Total Calories Consumed:_____
VS　　　　**Difference**
Total Calories Burned:_____

Personal Training Log

WEIGHT TRAINING

Date:_____ Phase:_____

Start:_____ Finish:_____ Duration:_____

Day:_____ Warm Up:_____

EXERCISE	SET X REPS X WEIGHT @ TEMPO
1.	___X___X_____@__/__/__
	___X___X_____@__/__/__
	___X___X_____@__/__/__
	___X___X_____@__/__/__
	___X___X_____@__/__/__
2.	___X___X_____@__/__/__
	___X___X_____@__/__/__
	___X___X_____@__/__/__
	___X___X_____@__/__/__
	___X___X_____@__/__/__
3.	___X___X_____@__/__/__
	___X___X_____@__/__/__
	___X___X_____@__/__/__
	___X___X_____@__/__/__
	___X___X_____@__/__/__
4.	___X___X_____@__/__/__
	___X___X_____@__/__/__
	___X___X_____@__/__/__
	___X___X_____@__/__/__
	___X___X_____@__/__/__
5.	___X___X_____@__/__/__
	___X___X_____@__/__/__
	___X___X_____@__/__/__
	___X___X_____@__/__/__
	___X___X_____@__/__/__
6.	___X___X_____@__/__/__
	___X___X_____@__/__/__
	___X___X_____@__/__/__
	___X___X_____@__/__/__
	___X___X_____@__/__/__
7.	___X___X_____@__/__/__
	___X___X_____@__/__/__
	___X___X_____@__/__/__
	___X___X_____@__/__/__
	___X___X_____@__/__/__
8.	___X___X_____@__/__/__
	___X___X_____@__/__/__
	___X___X_____@__/__/__
	___X___X_____@__/__/__
	___X___X_____@__/__/__
9.	___X___X_____@__/__/__
	___X___X_____@__/__/__
	___X___X_____@__/__/__
	___X___X_____@__/__/__
	___X___X_____@__/__/__

3

CARDIO SESSION #1

TIME:_____

ACTIVITY:_____

DURATION:_____ LEVEL_____

DISTANCE:_____

CALORIES BURNED:_____

ACTIVITY PULSE RATE:_____bpm

RECOVERY PULSE RATE:_____bpm

DIFFERENCE:

DAILY SLEEP TRACKER

TIME TO BED:_____

TIME UP:_____

HOURS OF SLEEP:_____

COMMENTS:_____

DAILY AB TRACKER

EXERCISE	SET X REPS X WGT
1._____	___X___X___
2._____	___X___X___
3._____	___X___X___
4._____	___X___X___
5._____	___X___X___

FITNESS CLASS
(or any physical activity-walk, jog, squash)

START:_____ FINISH:_____

TYPE:_____

INSTRUCTOR:_____

ESTIMATE OF
CALORIES BURNED:

COMMENTS:_____

CARDIO SESSION #2

TIME:_____

ACTIVITY:_____

DURATION:_____ LEVEL_____

DISTANCE:_____

CALORIES BURNED:_____

ACTIVITY PULSE RATE:_____bpm

RECOVERY PULSE RATE:_____bpm

DIFFERENCE:_____

COMMENTS:_____

TOTAL CALORIES
BURNED TODAY:

Daily Nutrition Tracking

NUTRITION	Points Goal	CAL option	PROT grams	FAT grams	CARB grams
Meal #1 – Time: H₂O____Cups(L)					
Meal #2 – Time: H₂O____Cups(L)					
Meal #3 – Time: H₂O____Cups(L)					
Meal #4 – Time: H₂O____Cups(L)					
Meal #5 – Time: H₂O____Cups(L)					
Meal #6 Time: H₂O____Cups(L)					
Food Point Total For Today:					
Difference (Goal Points Minus Actual Points)					
Daily Totals: (Add up each nutrient column. Convert each to calories. Add all and enter in "Total Calories")			g	g	g
Conversion To Calories Multiply Total Grams of **Pro X 4** = Calories / Multiply Total Grams of **Carb X 4**=Calories / Multiply Total Grams of **Fat X 9** = Calories	**Total Calories**		cal	cal	cal
Daily Percentages: (Divide total calories of each nutrient by the Total Number of Calories)			%	%	%
Total Calories Consumed:_____ VS *Difference* **Total Calories Burned:** _____					

3

Personal Training Log

WEIGHT TRAINING

Date:_____ Phase:_____

Start:_____ Finish:_____ Duration:_____

Day:_____ Warm Up:_____

EXERCISE	SET X REPS X WEIGHT @ TEMPO
1.	___X___X_____@__/__/__
	___X___X_____@__/__/__
	___X___X_____@__/__/__
	___X___X_____@__/__/__
	___X___X_____@__/__/__
2.	___X___X_____@__/__/__
	___X___X_____@__/__/__
	___X___X_____@__/__/__
	___X___X_____@__/__/__
	___X___X_____@__/__/__
3.	___X___X_____@__/__/__
	___X___X_____@__/__/__
	___X___X_____@__/__/__
	___X___X_____@__/__/__
	___X___X_____@__/__/__
4.	___X___X_____@__/__/__
	___X___X_____@__/__/__
	___X___X_____@__/__/__
	___X___X_____@__/__/__
	___X___X_____@__/__/__
5.	___X___X_____@__/__/__
	___X___X_____@__/__/__
	___X___X_____@__/__/__
	___X___X_____@__/__/__
	___X___X_____@__/__/__
6.	___X___X_____@__/__/__
	___X___X_____@__/__/__
	___X___X_____@__/__/__
	___X___X_____@__/__/__
	___X___X_____@__/__/__
7.	___X___X_____@__/__/__
	___X___X_____@__/__/__
	___X___X_____@__/__/__
	___X___X_____@__/__/__
	___X___X_____@__/__/__
8.	___X___X_____@__/__/__
	___X___X_____@__/__/__
	___X___X_____@__/__/__
	___X___X_____@__/__/__
	___X___X_____@__/__/__
9.	___X___X_____@__/__/__
	___X___X_____@__/__/__
	___X___X_____@__/__/__
	___X___X_____@__/__/__
	___X___X_____@__/__/__

CARDIO SESSION #1

TIME:_____

ACTIVITY:_____

DURATION:_____ LEVEL_____

DISTANCE:_____

CALORIES BURNED:_____

ACTIVITY PULSE RATE:_____bpm

RECOVERY PULSE RATE:_____bpm

DIFFERENCE:

DAILY SLEEP TRACKER

TIME TO BED:_____

TIME UP:_____

HOURS OF SLEEP:_____

COMMENTS:_____

DAILY AB TRACKER

EXERCISE	SET X REPS X WGT
1._____	___X___X____
2._____	___X___X____
3._____	___X___X____
4._____	___X___X____
5._____	___X___X____

FITNESS CLASS

(or any physical activity-walk, jog, squash)

START:_____ FINISH:_____

TYPE:_____

INSTRUCTOR:_____

ESTIMATE OF
CALORIES BURNED:

COMMENTS:_____

CARDIO SESSION #2

TIME:_____

ACTIVITY:_____

DURATION:_____ LEVEL_____

DISTANCE:_____

CALORIES BURNED:_____

ACTIVITY PULSE RATE:_____bpm

RECOVERY PULSE RATE:_____bpm

DIFFERENCE:_____

COMMENTS:_____

TOTAL CALORIES
BURNED TODAY:

3

NUTRITION	Points Goal	CAL *option*	PROT *grams*	FAT *grams*	CARB *grams*
Meal #1 – Time: H₂O____Cups(L)					
Meal #2 – Time: H₂O____Cups(L)					
Meal #3 – Time: H₂O____Cups(L)					
Meal #4 – Time: H₂O____Cups(L)					
Meal #5 – Time: H₂O____Cups(L)					
Meal #6 – Time: H₂O____Cups(L)					
Food Point Total For Today:					
Difference (Goal Points Minus Actual Points)					
Daily Totals: (Add up each nutrient column. Convert each to calories. Add all and enter in "Total Calories")			g	g	g
Conversion To Calories Multiply Total Grams of **Pro X 4** = Calories / Multiply Total Grams of **Carb X 4** = Calories / Multiply Total Grams of **Fat X 9** = Calories	**Total Calories**		cal	cal	cal
Daily Percentages: (Divide total calories of each nutrient by the Total Number of Calories)			___%	___%	___%

Total Calories Consumed:_____
                    VS   **Difference**
Total Calories Burned: _____

3

Progress Evaluation

Did you meet your goals for this cycle?   Yes ☐   No ☐

If not, what prevented you from reaching your goals?

_____

_____

_____

_____

State the positive changes that occurred during this cycle even if you didn't meet all your goals:

_____

_____

_____

_____

What do you plan to do differently during the next cycle?

_____

_____

_____

Personal Trainers/Teachers Evaluation

_____

_____

_____

_____

_____

_____

_____